FEMTOSECOND LASER-ASSISTED KERATOPLASTY

FEMTOSECOND LASER-ASSISTED KERATOPLASTY

Editor

Jorge L Alió MD PhD
Professor and Chairman
Department of Ophthalmology
Miguel Hernandez University, Medical School
President, Vissum Corporation
Alicante, Spain

Associate Editors

Alfredo Vega MD PhD
Cornea Transplantation Unit
Vissum-Instituto Oftalmologico de Alicante
Alicante, Spain

Felipe Soria MD
Cornea Transplantation Unit
Vissum-Instituto Oftalmologico de Alicante
Alicante, Spain

JAYPEE BROTHERS MEDICAL PUBLISHERS (P) LTD

New Delhi • London • Philadelphia • Panama

Jaypee Brothers Medical Publishers (P) Ltd

Headquarters

Jaypee Brothers Medical Publishers (P) Ltd
4838/24, Ansari Road, Daryaganj
New Delhi 110 002, India
Phone: +91-11-43574357
Fax: +91-11-43574314
Email: jaypee@jaypeebrothers.com

Overseas Offices

J.P. Medical Ltd
83 Victoria Street, London
SW1H 0HW (UK)
Phone: +44-2031708910
Fax: +02-03-0086180
Email: info@jpmedpub.com

Jaypee-Highlights Medical Publishers Inc.
City of Knowledge, Bld. 237, Clayton
Panama City, Panama
Phone: + 507-301-0496
Fax: + 507-301-0499
Email: cservice@jphmedical.com

Jaypee Medical Inc.
The Bourse
111 South Independence Mall East
Suite 835, Philadelphia, PA 19106, USA
Phone: + 267-519-9789
Email: joe.rusko@jaypeebrothers.com

Jaypee Brothers Medical Publishers (P) Ltd
17/1-B Babar Road, Block-B, Shaymali
Mohammadpur, Dhaka-1207
Bangladesh
Mobile: +08801912003485
Email: jaypeedhaka@gmail.com

Jaypee Brothers Medical Publishers (P) Ltd
Shorakhute, Kathmandu
Nepal
Phone: +00977-9841528578
Email: jaypee.nepal@gmail.com

Website: www.jaypeebrothers.com
Website: www.jaypeedigital.com

Inquiries for bulk sales may be solicited at: jaypee@jaypeebrothers.com

Femtosecond Laser-Assisted Keratoplasty

First Edition: 2013

ISBN : 978-93-5090-509-8

Printed at: Ajanta Offset & Packagings Ltd., New Delhi

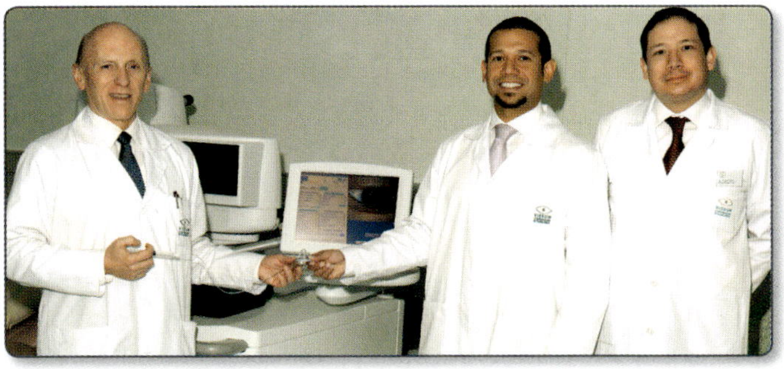

Dedicated to

Our families, who sacrifice their time
to make this project possible.
The time, dedication and excitement of a new project
like the femtosecond corneal grafting techniques
book competes always with the time
that we devote to our families
even though in our hearts
there is no time for anything other than for them.

Contributors

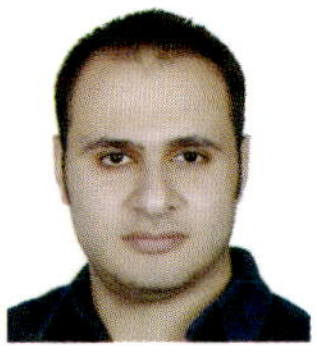

Ahmed A Abdou MD PhD
Clinical Research Fellow
Vissum Corporation
Alicante, Spain

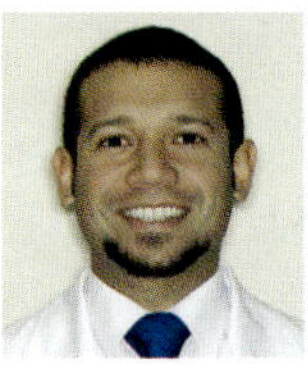

Alfredo Vega MD PhD
Cornea Transplantation Unit
Vissum-Instituto Oftalmologico de Alicante
Alicante, Spain

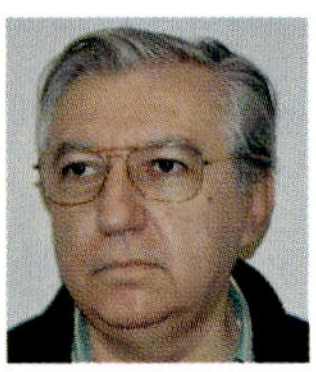

Antonio Fimia PhD
Professor
Departamento de Ciencia de los Materiales
Óptica y Tecnología Electrónica
Universidad Miguel Hernández de Elche
Alicante, Spain

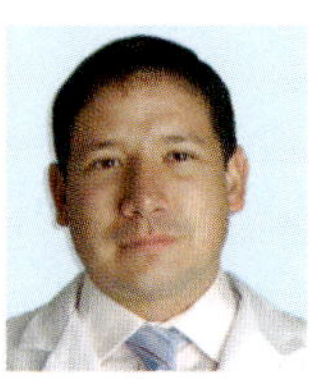

Felipe Soria MD
Cornea Transplantation Unit
Vissum-Instituto Oftalmologico de Alicante
Alicante, Spain

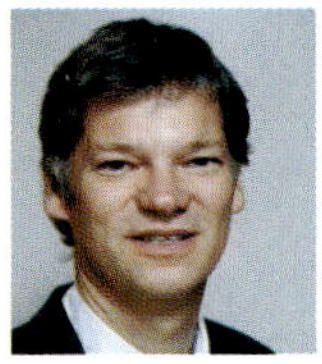

Georg Gerten MD
Consulting Ophthalmologist
Augenklinik am Neumarkt
Köln, Germany

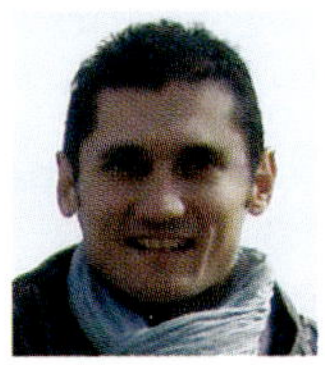

Jean-Louis Bourges MD PhD FEBO
Associate Professor
Sorbonne Paris Cité University, Paris
Descartes Faculty of Medicine, Department of Ophthalmology, Hôtel-Dieu, APHP
Paris, France

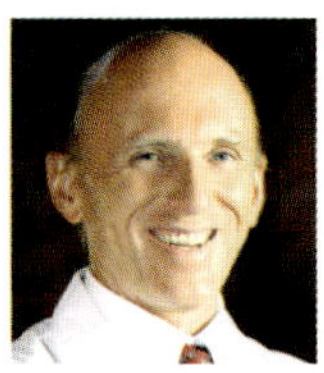

Jorge L Alió MD PhD
Professor and Chairman
Department of Ophthalmology
Miguel Hernandez University, Medical School
President, Vissum Corporation
Alicante, Spain

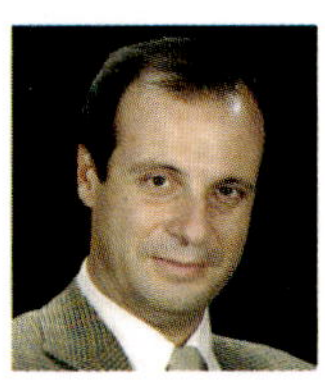

Juan Alvarez de Toledo MD
Centro de Oftalmología Barraquer
Barcelona, Spain

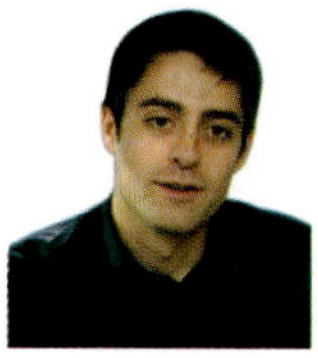

Juan Gabriel Ortiz MSc MBA
Telecommunication Engineering
Development Director, IMEX, Spain

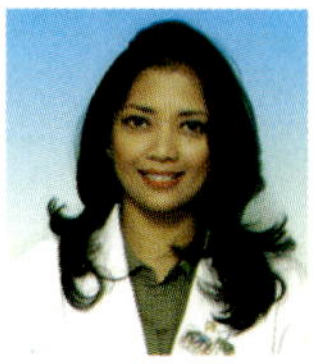

María F de la Paz MD
Centro de Oftalmología Barraquer
Barcelona, Spain

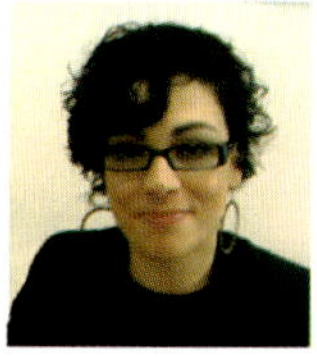

M Gomariz PhD
Professor
Departamento de Ciencia de los Materiales
Óptica y Tecnología Electrónica
Universidad Miguel Hernández de Elche
Alicante, Spain

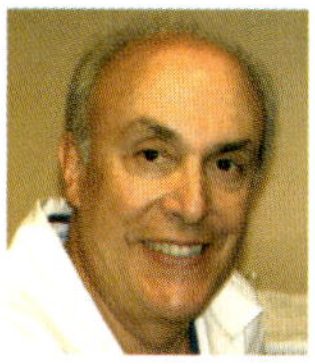

Perry S Binder MS MD
Clinical Professor
Gavin Herbert Eye Institute
University of California
Irvine, California, USA

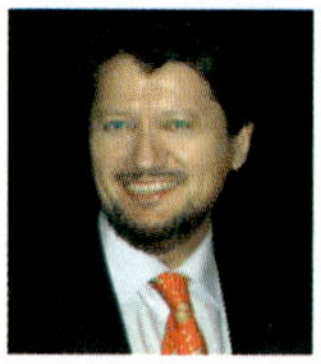

Rafael I Barraquer-Compte MD PhD
Centro de Oftalmología Barraquer
Barcelona, Spain

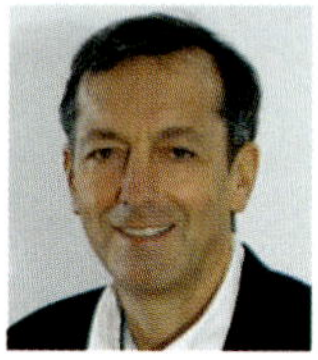

Tobias Neuhann MD
Clinical Director
Augenklinik der Ludwig-Maximilians-Universität
Muenchen, Germany

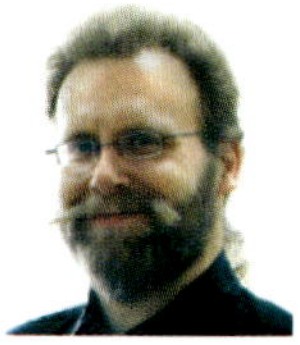

Uwe Oberheide PhD
Augenklinik am Neumarkt
Köln, Germany

Preface

This book is dedicated to those corneal surgeons specifically interested in corneal transplantation techniques and who are looking for its improvement by the innovation created by recent progress in the technology applicable to corneal grafting surgery. One of the most important steps forward, which recently has fostered and promoted the development of corneal grafting in terms of better standards of quality, is indeed, the use of femtosecond lasers to create better cutting profiles to match donor and recipient corneas promoting better outcomes.

Why have we felt that this book is necessary? In general, corneal grafting techniques are affected by many variables, biological, immunological, biomechanical, surgical and technological, which make this procedure intrinsically variable. The variability of the outcomes affects not only the visual and refractive outcomes but also the biological performance of the tissues affected by the graft and by the surgical trauma and, overall, the visual recovery of the patient. It is our experience that the use of femtosecond lasers has improved many of these variables making corneal grafting surgery a better and more controllable technique with better outcomes. In this early moment in which femtosecond lasers are being applied more and more to corneal surgery, such information is disperse and scarce. This book aims to make this recent information accessible to the many surgeons worldwide interested in this topic.

Femtosecond laser energy used at the cornea level involves specific issues, which have to be understood. This has indeed created a revolution in corneal surgery, which is at this moment at the beginning. The application of femtosecond laser not only to corneal refractive surgery (flap creation, intrastromal lenticule creation and precise optical profiles for its extraction to correct myopia), but also to other procedures, such as tunnel creation for intracorneal rings and segment implantations, pockets for intracorneal inlays and rings, astigmatic incisions, cataract surgery incisions and others are clear examples of the impressive usefulness of a technology, which has arrived to stay and to change our way to understand and use surgical instruments in corneal surgery. Indeed, femtosecond laser is widening the indications of corneal surgery, as the flexibility of profiles and the quality of femtosecond laser created cuts jointly with the minimal invasiveness of the procedure, have fostered new creativity in innovative corneal surgeons.

This book aims to instruct the corneal surgeon in the ways in which femtosecond lasers can be used for corneal grafting surgery. To do this properly, we have invited selected opinion leader surgeons with extensive experience in this innovative technology and who use different technologies to offer their practical approaches for corneal lamellar grafts, penetrating grafts and alternative lamellar graft techniques, such as corneal excision. As the level of evidence still reported is not high, but it is more about the surgical practicality and personal experience of such innovative surgeons, this book approaches this surgical technique and the femtosecond technology from a practical point of view. The reader will find the ways in which the technologies can be used, how to use the different elements involved in the procedure properly, such as artificial anterior chambers and a comment about the level of evidence that we have at this moment on the use of femtosecond laser as a better technology to create the corneal donor and recipient cutting interfaces for the purpose of improving refractive visual and clinical outcomes. In this respect, it is the first book on this technology and topic to be published so far.

We hope the reader will enjoy the different chapters of this book devoted entirely to corneal grafting surgery assisted by femtosecond lasers. As evidence of better outcomes increases, the use of this technology in corneal surgery will experience a tremendous development in the future. This book is the first one on the topic of femtosecond-assisted corneal transplantation techniques and will probably be followed by others in the future on this emerging and most interesting area of ophthalmic surgery.

ADVANTAGES OF FEMTOSECOND LASER-ASSISTED KERATOPLASTY (FLAK) OVER CONVENTIONAL GRAFT SURGERY

The capability of femtosecond laser energy to create different profiles with a controlled level of biological interaction and minimal tissue trauma has provided a new possibility for corneal grafting surgeons. Not only are the minimal aggressiveness of the procedure due to the very light and controllable light tissue interaction but also for the speed of the profiles created, femtosecond lasers a perfect blade for the purpose of corneal grafting surgery. Their precision and capability to create a better donor-host interaction promoting a faster wound healing process is obvious, but also unsolved issues, such as the sutures necessary to fix the donor to the recipient and the timing during which these stitches have to be placed is indeed affected by the procedure. The main advantages that we, as corneal surgeons, find for the use of femtosecond laser in corneal grafting surgery over conventional cutting techniques are given in Table 1.

Femtosecond laser side cuts are more precise and regular. This is not surprising because the femtosecond profiles are created under controlled conditions, which is something that never happens in manual trephination techniques. Variables, such as the intraocular pressure, trephination angle, eye position among others, are avoided by the controlled position of the eye created by the suction ring and the conditions of application of femtosecond lasers. The risk of penetration when performing full graft trephination as happens in manual techniques does not occur in femtosecond laser-assisted penetrating keratoplasty. First of all, the cuts are not total; and secondly, they are open in the operating room under a microscope without the risk of penetrating the eye, creating injury to the iris, crystalline lens or other intraocular structures.

By definition, this capability of controlling the cut and the profile with less potential surgical trauma makes the perfect environment for an adequately precise donor-recipient size matching. Traditionally, mismatching has been used in donor-recipient sizing due to the lack of confidence in the adequate apposition of the cut tissue. On the contrary, with femtosecond lasers we do have this precision and as the matching should be perfect. The consequence of this is a much more controllable refractive outcome, probably less astigmatism and better anatomical evolution. In penetrating corneal graft techniques, the damage to the donor corneal endothelium was always expected. This comes from the fact of the relatively traumatic cutting maneuvers that had to be performed from the endothelial side under uncontrolled conditions. In femtosecond laser surgery, the donor tissue is cut even in penetrating grafts in a closed environment, thanks to the use of the artificial anterior chamber. The much more physiological conditions of femtosecond laser trephination make it less traumatic for the corneal endothelium with a far better expectation of preserving its integrity.

One of the most interesting and probably important issues related to femtosecond laser side cuts both in penetrating and non-penetrating corneal procedures is the potential for customization of the cutting pattern. From case to case and procedure to procedure, the pattern profile could be more convenient in one or another cutting profile alternative, which was impossible to be made before with the manual trephination techniques. These profiles can make the donor tissue and the recipient to be adjusted as a cork enters into the bottle. Indeed, the optimized position of the donor and recipient tissues guarantees a more stable anatomy and potentially simplifies the use of sutures or other methods to join the two tissues. This cutting pattern, being more complex, offers an increased donor-host interface with an improved tissue interaction, which promotes better wound healing. This will improve the short-term evolution of the grafted eye, probably making the extraction of the sutures shorter or the fixation techniques that have been used to join the tissue and promotes faster wound healing inducing a much more stable evolution of the graft. Most probably, this capability to control the profiles of the side cuts, an almost perfect donor-recipient sizing and faster wound healing should lead to less induction of surgically induced astigmatism both on a short-term and a long-term basis. All corneal surgeons know how unpredictable the post-graft astigmatism is as so many variables are involved, particularly one of the most important being the sutures, which cannot be avoided today. It is, in my opinion, an expected step in the future to have alternatives to fixate the donor tissue to the recipient avoiding the use of sutures, thanks to the use of different bioadhesives or other alternative methods of fixation. Overall speaking, these advantages would promote a shorter visual rehabilitation time, with less unpredictable refractive outcomes and a shorter follow-up period for the patients. If all this is true, a stronger and more stable corneal

Table 1: Advantages of femtosecond laser-assisted keratoplasty over conventional corneal graft surgery
1. More precise and regular cuts
2. No risk of injury for intraocular structures
3. Perfect donor-recipient size matching
4. Less injury to donor endothelium
5. Customization of the cutting pattern, possible from case to case
6. More donor-host tissue interaction promoting better wound healing
7. Potentially less induction of surgically induced astigmatism
8. Probably shorter visual rehabilitation time
9. Stronger and probably more stable wounds with earlier suture removal

wound healing is created, with fewer refractive surprises, less corneal irregularity, and shorter rehabilitation time, we would end in an immensely improved corneal graft outcome.

In today's surgical environment, we should demand a new surgical technique to confirm reliability, evidence that expected outcomes are better than before, with fewer complications both in severity and frequency, and capability to prevent previous complications by better planning. We need and we want to have fewer surgical surprises and a balanced cost-benefit ratio. So far, and throughout the chapters of this book, we have realized that today even though the evidence is limited, we have all these items accomplished.

Jorge L Alió

Contents

Introduction

Perry S Binder

An ophthalmologist who began refractive surgery in the last 5 years might not understand the impact, the femtosecond laser has had on anterior segment surgery. But for those who performed refractive corneal surgery prior to 1999, they can deeply appreciate the impact of femtosecond surgery on almost everything they do today.

The idea of using a femtosecond laser for ophthalmic surgery came from a resident in ophthalmology, Dr Ronald Kurtz who observed minimal retinal damage to a laser researcher who accidentally received a femtosecond laser beam injury to their retina. The serendipity of subsequently meeting a femtosecond laser specialist, Dr Tibor Juhasz a short time thereafter at a femtosecond laser conference led to the collaboration and development of the IntraLase Corporation. For those readers interested in the physics that led to the development of the anterior segment femtosecond laser, please read these selected references.[1-5]

The initial goal for using a femtosecond laser for corneal surgery was to remove a contact lens shape (lenticule) from the center of the corneal stroma (without cutting Bowman's layer) to change the anterior corneal curvature and thereby the refractive error.[4] In the few years preceding the formation of the IntraLase Corporation, the only laser available for reshaping the cornea was the picosecond laser developed by ISL Corporation. An example of their surgical procedure was presented before the American Academy of Ophthalmology in the fall of 1993 by Arturo Chayet.[6,7] Unfortunately, the slow speed and large cavitation bubbles presented this technology from accomplishing this goal. Today, this same procedure has reached the clinical level as the SMILE procedure performed on the Zeiss VisuMax femtosecond laser.

Many of the staff of the ISL Corporation were experienced femtosecond laser technicians. Everyone went on to develop their own variation of femtosecond laser technology. During a meeting at the fledgling of the IntraLase Corporation, doctors Kurtz and Juhasz asked the question "if we cannot change the corneal curvature with our laser technology what else can we do with it?" Someone suggested why not use it to create a corneal flap? The first LASIK procedure performed on a sighted human eye was on September 3, 1999 in Budapest, Hungary by surgeon Dr Imola Ratkay Traub.[8] That laser had an engine speed of 2 kHz, which took approximately 3 minutes to create a 9 mm flap. For those experienced femtosecond laser, surgeons who are reading this introduction, you will be interested to know that the raster energy exceeded 4 μJ and the sidecut energy exceeded 6 μJ. The spot and line separation was greater than 14 × 14 μ.

At about the same time, the Femtec femtosecond laser was being used for early corneal transplantation studies, but at that time in the early 2000s there were no other femtosecond laser companies involved in corneal surgery.[9,10] In 2000, the IntraLase Corporation increased the engine speed to 6 kHz and distributed three beta versions to doctors Dishler, Slade, and Nordan.[11] In early 2001, the IntraLase Corporation received a 510 K approval from the US FDA to create LASIK flaps and began selling their first clinical version whose engine speed was 10 kHz.

The first mechanical microkeratomes were manufactured and distributed by Steinway instruments under the direction of Dr Jose Barraquer. Subsequently, the Chiron Corporation through the advice of Dr Luis Ruiz developed and distributed the first Automated Corneal shaper (ACS).[12] There then followed several generations and improvements in mechanical microkeratomes so that by 2002, at least eight different mechanical microkeratome companies were selling instrumentation. In 2000, I personally owned six microkeratomes and had served as medical director for three of the companies. When the IntraLase Corporation first contacted our company and presented their technology, I was skeptical because I was very pleased with my mechanical microkeratome results. Nevertheless, we were among the first to purchase this new technology. In March 2002, I performed my first procedure on the 10 kHz laser which took 97 seconds to create a 9 mm flap. The raster energy was 3 μJ, the sidecut energy was 6 μJ, and the spot and line separation was 12 × 12 μ. After measuring the central thickness of 30 flaps, I realized the potential of this new technology. I immediately called Dr Kurtz and told him I loved the technology and wanted to be his Medical Director. I have been in that position ever since and am currently with Abbott Medical Optics who purchased the IntraLase Corporation in 2008.

Between 2002 and 2008, the IntraLase Corporation improved its hardware and software to not only increase speed and efficiency of flap creation, but to add additional software modules to allow the placement of intracorneal rings,[13] to create arcuate incisions within the cornea,[14] to perform lamellar corneal transplants,[15] and in my opinion, the most important addition was the software that allowed surgeons to perform shaped lamellar and penetrating corneal transplants—the IntraLase Enabled Keratoplasty (IEK) software.[16] In 2012, Abbott Medical Optics, the company that purchased the IntraLase Corporation in 2008, received additional 510 K approval for penetrating and intrastromal arcuate incisions as well as the creation of clear corneal incisions to assist cataract surgery.

Following the introduction of the IntraLase technology, several other femtosecond laser companies were developed.[17] Through improvements in technology and the ingenuity of engineers and surgeons, many new anterior segment corneal procedures have been developed so that today it is not inconceivable for a surgeon to apply femtosecond laser technology in circumstances where they previously used a metal or diamond blade. The technology has now advanced beyond the cornea to permit peripheral limbal surgery, and more recently surgery on the crystalline lens to remove the capsule and to fragment the nucleus.[18,19] As the reader will discover in this book there are now over 20 anterior segment applications that have been published or presented that utilize femtosecond laser technology for anterior segment surgery.[20-22]

In 2001, 100% of LASIK flap creation was performed by mechanical microkeratomes in the United States. In 2012, over 75% of LASIK procedures are performed with femtosecond laser technology in the United States with a similar increase in market penetration outside the United States. The advent of femtosecond laser technology has stimulated the improvement in mechanical microkeratomes so that the current, fifth-generation instrumentation is safer and more predictable than ever before. Even today there remain some staunch mechanical microkeratome users who consider their instrumentation's capabilities of producing predictable LASIK flaps similar to those of femtosecond lasers.[23] Even if we assume that the studies are correct, one must not lose sight of the fact that mechanical microkeratomes still require the use of a blade. Because of the hardware used to connect the microkeratome to the globe, the creation of flap dimensions are dependent upon blade quality (quality of cut, thinner flaps for the mate eye, flap thickness dependent upon blade oscillation and translation, corneal curvature, corneal thickness, intraocular pressure). More importantly, mechanical microkeratomes are designed to create flaps whereas femtosecond lasers are much more than a mechanical microkeratome as they can create procedures that neither a microkeratome nor a diamond blade can create.

In the coming decade we will see additional applications of femtosecond technology within Ophthalmology, such as glaucoma procedures, scleral surgery, iris surgery and vitreous surgery. Even today femtosecond laser technology is being used to perform high resolution anatomic studies[24] and to perform individual cell surgery that could ultimately lead to selective nerve transection or blood vessel surgery. Laser engine speeds will increase to allow even closer spot and line separations for improved quality of tissue resection while permitting increased speeds of procedures with lower laser pulse energies that will decrease adjacent morphologic damage. Improvements in the software and the user interfaces will ultimately lead to voice control and integration between diagnostic instrumentation and the femtosecond laser so that is not inconceivable that individualized corneal flaps and other surgical procedures can be created based on patients' individual ocular and orbital anatomy and refractive errors. It is expected that the femtosecond laser application for cataract surgery will ultimately become the standard of care overcurrent ultrasound procedures. Femtosecond laser surgery will spur the development and application of new ophthalmic technologies, for example, the creation of an intracorneal pocket[25] to allow the implantation of corneal inlays for the correction of presbyopia. The same pockets can serve as a reservoir for antibiotics or for riboflavin is just another potential improvement for collagen crosslinking. It is not inconceivable that human corneal tissue or synthetic corneal tissue can be implanted in these pockets to increase corneal thickness or to modify refractive errors. The applications of anterior segment femtosecond surgery will only be limited by our imagination.

REFERENCES

1. Juhasz T, Kastis GA, Suárez C, et al. Time-resolved observations of shock waves and cavitation bubbles generated by femtosecond laser pulses in corneal tissue and water. Lasers Surg Med. 1996;19(1):23-31.
2. Loesel FH, Niemz MH, Billie JF, et al. Laser induced optical breakdown on hard and soft tissues and its dependence on the pulse duration. Experiment and model. IEEE J Quantum Electronics. 1996;32:1717-22.
3. Noack J, Vogel A. Laser-induced plasma formation in water at nanosecond to femtosecond time scales: calculation of thresholds, absorption coefficients and energy density. IEEE J Quantum Electron. 1999;35:1156-67.
4. Heisterkamp A, Mamom T, Drommer W, et al. Photodisruption with ultrashort laser pulses for intrastromal refractive surgery. Laser Physics. 2003;13:743-8.
5. Vogel A, Noack J. Mechanism of femtosecond laser nanosurgery of cells and tissue. Appl Phys B. 2005;81:1015.
6. Juhasz T, Hu XH, Turi L, et al. Dynamics of shock waves and cavitation bubbles generated by picosecond laser pulses in corneal tissue and water. Lasers in Surgery and Medicine. 1994;15:91-8.

7. Juhasz T, Speaker M, Habib M, et al. Refractive effects of myopic intrastromal ablation of the cat cornea with the ND:YLF picosecond laser. Invest Ophthalmol Vis Sci. 1996.
8. Ratkay-Traub I, Juhasz T, Horvath C, et al. Ultra-Short Pulse (Femtosecond) Laser Surgery. Ophthalmol Clin North Am. 2000;14(2):347-55.
9. Lubatschowski H, Maatz G, Rudolph M, et al. Application of ultrashort laser pulses for intrastromal refractive surgery. Graefes Arch Clin Exp Ophthalmol. 2000;238(1):33-9.
10. Jonas J. Lamellar femtosecond laser keratoplasty with conical incisions and positional spikes. Graefes Arch Clin Exp Ophthalmol. 2003;241(9):781.
11. Nordan LT, Slade SG, Baker RN, et al. Femtosecond Laser Flap Creation for laser in situ keratomileusis. Six month follow-up of intitial U.S. clinical series. J Refract Surg. 2003;19(1):8-14.
12. Ruiz L, Slade SG, Updegraff SA. In: Salz J (Ed). Excimer Myopic Keratomelusis: Bogota Experience in Corneal Laser Surgery. St. Louis: Mosby-Year Book Inc; 1995. p. 195.
13. Ertan A, Bahadir M. Topography-guided vertical implantation of Intacs using a femtosecond laser for the treatement of keratoconus. J Cat Refr Surg. 2007;33(1):148-51.
14. Bahar I, Levinger E, Kaiserman I, et al. IntraLase-enabled astigmatic keratotomy for postkeratoplasty astigmatism. Am J Ophthalmol. 2008;146(6):897-904.
15. Sarayba MA, Maguen E, Salz J, et al. Femtosecond laser keratome creation of partial thickness donor corneal buttons for lamellar keratoplasty. J Refract Surg. 2007;23(1):58-65.
16. Steinert RF, Ignacio TS, Sarayba MA. "Top Hat"-shaped penetrating keratoplasty using the femtosecond laser. Am J Ophthalmol. 2007;143(4):689-91.
17. Lubatschowski H. Overview of commercially available femtosecond lasers in refractive surgery. J Refract Surg. 2008;24(1):S102-7.
18. Nagy ZZ, Kránitz K, Takacs AI, et al. Comparison of Intraocular Lens Decentration Parameters After Femtosecond and Manual Capsulotomies. J Refract Surg. 2011;27(8):564-9.
19. Bali SJ, Hodge C, Lawless M, et al. Early Experience with the Femtosecond Laser for Cataract Surgery. Ophthalmology. 2012;119(5):891-9.
20. Kima P, Sutton GL, Rootman DS. Applications of the femtosecond laser in corneal refractive surgery. Curr Opin Ophthalmol. 2011;22(4)238-44.
21. Shousha MA, Yoo SH. New therapeutic modalities in femtosecond laser-assisted corneal surgery. Int Ophthalmol Clin. 2010;50(3):149-60.
22. Kullman G, Pineda II R. Alternative applications of the femtosecond laser in Ophthalmology. Sem Ophthalmol. 2010;25(5-6):256-64.
23. Paschalis EI, Labiris G, Aristeidou AP, et al. Laser in situ keratomileusis flap-thickness predictability with a pendular microkeratome. J Cat Refr Surg. 2011;37(12):2160-6.
24. Winkler M, Chai D, Kriling S, et al. Nonlinear Optical Macroscopic Assessment of 3-D Corneal Collagen Organization and Axial Biomechanics. Invest Ophthalmol VIs Sci. 2011;52(12):8818-27.
25. Binder PS. Software for Intracorneal Pockets. Invest Ophthalmol Vis Sci. ARVO Abstracts, 2010.

Chapter

1

Femtosecond Laser Corneal Tissue Interaction

Antonio Fimia, M Gomariz

CHAPTER OUTLINE

Interaction processes between light energy and ocular tissues
Femtosecond laser corneal surgery systems

- Description of the most important characteristics of laser systems currently available for ocular femtosecond assisted surgery with special focus in femtosecond assisted corneal surgery.

Light-Tissue Interaction

- Sequence of events happening during the irradiation process: how it happens photodisruption, as a consequence of the interaction between femtosecond pulses and ocular tissues.
- Physical processes involved in the propagation of an ultrashort laser pulse into corneal tissue. Relationship among energy levels, time and repetition in the development of the process.
- Importance of internal thermic action in corneal tissue due to laser irradiation with high repetition rate frequency.

Future Directions

- Improvement will be related to the development of new technologies to make the process more efficient. Lasers will be more compact and smaller in size, less costly and with variable optical apertures to be compatible with the use of femtosecond technology in different ocular tissues, particularly in the anterior segment structures of the eye.

INTRODUCTION

Since the advent of the laser in the sixties, many clinical applications have appeared in the field of ophthalmology, in fact we can say that there is a clear parallelism between the progress in the technology and manufacturing of lasers and their respective applications in ophthalmology.[1,2]

Moreover, their application in the area of ophthalmology has been subject to the study of light-tissue interaction processes, processes that have initially been linked to nonlinear optics and with the introduction of lasers with a short-pulsed temporal duration, have allowed intensities per unit area above 10^{11} W/cm^2 to be reached. For this reason, models based on nonlinear optics for the analysis and justification of experimental results has been used.

Initially, the basic mechanism of interaction used was photocoagulation. That is to say the energy-focused generated an increase in the temperature in the irradiated area producing a process of coagulation. On the other hand, infrared radiation could also be applied resulting in a greater penetration of the tissue and a process of reducing the thickness of the tissue. These mechanisms are produced with continuous laser waves controlling irradiation times between a microsecond and second.

As a second development, they began using ultraviolet lasers with nanosecond pulse durations, which lead to photoablation processes. Laser-Assisted in Situ Keratomileusis (LASIK) and photorefractive keratectomy (PRK) surgery was the best known clinical consequence of this.[3]

From a historic point of view, the earlier works from the 1970s and 1980s to 2002 about the ultrashort laser pulse bioeffects has been analyzed in the Milestone series edited by Roach and Johnson. The nonlinear-induced phenomenon like self-focusing, laser-induced breakdown and nonlinear absorption that are observed in the ultrashort laser pulse bioeffects are presented and analyzed in the different papers selected by the editors. The classification of nonlinear effects, histology and safety give us excellent information about theoretical and experimental applications of laser technology for tissue modification by laser interaction.[1]

In 1974, Krasnov[2] introduced the Q-switched laser in process of interaction with ocular tissues for glaucoma and during the last decades many ophthalmologic surgery techniques have been applied to optimize human health care.

The first implementation studies focusing on the use of lasers with allows us to direct the laser beam in one direction and the second property allows us to concentrate on a small area of space with very high intensity. Pulses of less than a picosecond began in the late nineties, resulting in the process of photorupture. That is to say, processes which generate a mechanical rupture inside a tissue due to the creation of plasma.[4]

The general feature in all these processes was due to a technological development designed to have a greater local action of the interaction and a reduction of the unwanted effects, such as scattering and the thermal modification of the tissue structure near the irradiated area.

More recently, Juhasz (1999)[5,6] introduced near infrared femtosecond (fs) lasers in corneal surgery, as a result of the research project developed during the 1980s and 2000s by other authors in transparent materials.[7,8]

Recently, femtosecond lasers have been used for creating flaps in refractive surgery and other ophthalmic surgeries. Since the 2000s, this technological evolution process including pulse energy, laser repetition rate, wavelength, etc. have been analyzed and optimized in clinical systems.[2,9]

The aim of this chapter is to present, briefly, the main interaction process between ultrashort light pulses and cornea tissue. We will try to present this theoretical mechanism with diagrams and basic equations and define the most important parameters that are involved in the interaction process.

In Figure 1.1, we present a simple diagram which indicates the processes described above and in the table (attached) we present the different processes, laser characteristics and interaction times, according to the excellent book written by H Niemz.[3]

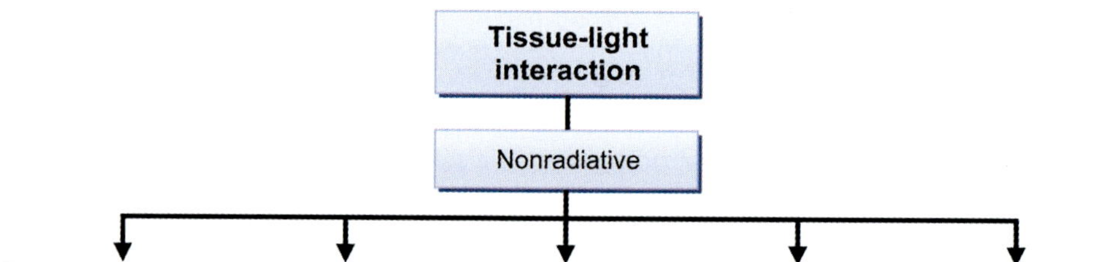

	Photochemical	Thermal	Photoablation	Plasma-induced ablation	Photodisruption
Fundamentals	Photosensitizer acting as catalyst	The temperature leads to a desired thermal effect, coagulation, vaporization and melting	Breaking of molecular bonds with UV photons	Ablation by ionizing plasma formation	Fragmentation and cutting tissue by mechanical forces
Lasers	Red dye laser diode	CO_2, Nd:YAG, Er:YAG, Ho, YAG	ArF, KrF, XeCl, XeF	Nd:YAG, ND:YLF, Ti: Sapphire	Solid-state lasers Nd: YAG, Nd:YLF, Ti: Sapphire
Pulse duration	1 s-CW	1 μs – 1ms	10–100 ns	100 fs – 500 ps	100 fs – 100 ns
Power densities (W/cm^2)	10^{-2}-S	$10–10^{6}$	$10^{7}–10^{10}$	$10^{11}–10^{13}$	$10^{11}–10^{16}$

Fig. 1.1: Non-radiative fundamental process in laser-tissue interaction (Neimz et al, 2003)[3]

INTERACTION PROCESSES IN MATERIALS WITH HIGH INTENSITIES

One of the key features of lasers, as we have comment, is that they are light sources with a high capacity for directionality and focalization. The first characteristic allows us to direct the laser beam in one direction and the second allows us to concentrate a very high intensity on a small area. Also, with ultrashort pulse time lasers it is possible to carry out nonlinear optical phenomena when interacting with transparent materials.[6] The photo rupture process is based on this conceptual basis.

The mechanisms, which are involved in the non-linear optical processes are based on the fact that, in the interaction zone of the beam with the medium, electric fields are generated with a value exceeding the value maintained in equilibrium the electron-nucleus interaction. This way, the atoms are fragmented; generating plasma whose first action is to modify the medium, thus, generating high temperature zones with the size of a micron in very short time, less than the thermal diffusion in the material.

Non-linear optical processes also have the possibility of modifying the refraction index of the material. In this case, the refraction index depends on the intensity so that a control on the intensity level applied to the material can lead us to control of the final index of refraction once the irradiation has been carried out.[10]

In this case, the mathematical equation, which allows us to evaluate the change in the refraction index is: $n = n_0 + n_1$ Here, n_0 is the refraction index of non-irradiated material and n_1 is a parameter characteristic of each material. A second effect caused by n_1 is the auto-focalization of the beam, which leads to an increase in the local action causing the material acts as a lens.

As mentioned before, a great number of free electrons are generated in the focalization area due to the action of the electric field generated causing the generation of plasma electrons, and consequently the process of photoionization.

If we consider the material as a semiconductor, the photoionization is based on the cooperation of various photons to excite the electrons of the atoms, which form the material in a way that they pass from the valence band to the conduction. This photoexcitation effect can be produced by multiphotonic or by a non-linear effect. The fact that either mechanism is produced depends on the Keldysh parameter, which reflects the influence of the different parameters involved in the irradiation and the material.

As a result, according to the intensity regime used, we can consider that different mechanisms generating the spatial rupture process of the material and also the speed of the photoionization which these mechanisms produce depends on the intensity and the multiphoton dispersion coefficient which characterizes these materials (Figs 1.2A and B).

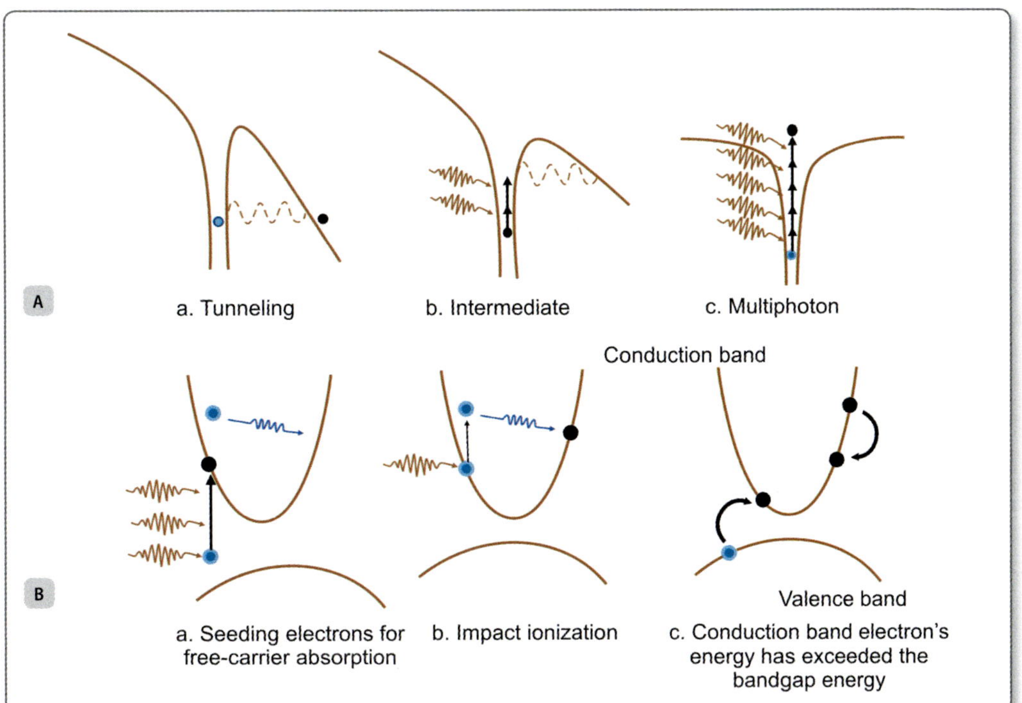

Figs 1.2A and B: (A) Schematic of tunneling, (a) intermediate (b) and multiphoton regimes (c) of high-intensity photoionization in an atom.[7] (B) Illustration of a multiphoton ionization (a) for seeding electrons for free-carrier absorption (b) followed by impact ionization (c) once de conduction band electrons energy has exceeded the band gap energy[11]

As we can see in Figure 1.2, the avalanche ionization is a two-step process. In the first step, electrons gain the energy from the electromagnetic field of the laser pulse, and after the electrons are dissociated by subsequent collisions with either atoms or ions.

For picosecond pulses multiphoton processes are not taken into account but with femtosecond pulses, multiphoton process might become significant.

Once the warm microplasm has been created, it expands at a supersonic speed creating "shockwaves", moving and breaking the area surrounding the material. As this process is produced adiabatically, it occurs in a time scale less than those of the thermal effects, the cutting effect is especially confined and therefore the thermal damage does not spread to the surrounding regions.

The shockwave, cavitation bubble and the pulse duration is decreased to femtosecond range. The shockwave pressure decreased from 7×10^8 Pa to 3×10^7 Pa in a radius of approximately 30 µm, while for picosecond pulses the radius was 200 µm.

It is evident that both the optical system used to focus on the tissue and the internal structure of the material being irradiated play a fundamental role for the adequate outcome of locally breaking the structure without damaging its surrounding.

A very important aspect in this process is the laser repetition frequency applied. If the frequency is within the kHz range, the mechanisms generated by each pulse are isolated and local. However, if the repetition frequencies applied are within the MHz range, the thermal effects are cumulative and different aspects should be considered, such as the irradiation time and the temporal pulse width.

Vogel et al.[13] extensively studied the influence of the intensity and frequency of repetition using water as well as polymeric materials and fabrics. It is important to remember that 75% of the cornea is water.

From 1999, studies began to appear which analyze in detail the different parameters and factors allowing internal cuts to be made in transparent in material.[13,14]

FEMTOSECOND SURGERY

As mentioned in the historical introduction, Juhasz[5] suggested using ultrashort pulse systems in ophthalmology by using them in cornea surgery with the IntraLaser system. In 2002, the FDA approved four surgical techniques as: corneal flap section for LASIK, keratomileusis, channel section for corneal implants and anterior lamellar corneal transplantation.[4]

All these techniques have been significantly evaluated and recently accepted for different clinical studies.

Lasers were initially used with kHz repetition frequencies and with wavelengths of 1050 nm, applying pulses of energy close to mJ. Table 1.1 shows some characteristics of these commercial systems as well as their most relevant data from a light-material interaction point of view.

As we can observed, all the clinical systems work with light repetition process and energies in µJ-mJ. Recently, there new techniques have been proposed that work with a light repetition rate in MHz and a very low pulse energy near to nJ.

As shown, all of them work with irradiated areas in order of micron and can act, in some cases, on curved surfaces. This technology is constantly being developed and current studies are planning on using lasers, which irradiate in 1550 nm. This will allow the work to be done by doubling the radiation frequency in the 777.5 nm,[9] wavelength near 800 nm in the systems mode-locked lasers by Ti: sapphire.

LIGHT-TISSUE INTERACTION

From an experimental point of view, the light-tissue study significantly differs from studies carried out in water and polymers. In the first place, the cornea, as well known, has a distinct layer structure and its spatial geometry has implications over the propagation and focusing of light beams. Moreover, each layer has a different composition of which a supposed 75% of the total volume of the cornea is water.

Table 1.1: Most important characteristics of laser systems currently available[9]

Name of system	*IntraLase fs*	*Femtec*	*Femto LDV*	*Visumax*
Laser system	Oscillator amplified	Femtec	Oscillator non-amplified	Oscillator fibre amplified
Wavelenght	1050 nm	1050 nm	1050 nm	1050 nm
Reflection rate	60 ó 150 kHz	40 ó 80 kHz	MHz	500 kHz
Pulse duration	400–800 fs	500–800 fs	200–300 fs	220–580 fs
Pulse energy	1 mJ	1 mJ	<<1 mJ	<<1 mJ
Spot size	A few µms	A few µms	<1 mm	1 µm
Applanation lens	Plane (Curved is possible)	Curved	Plane	Curved

As we can see in Figure 1.3, there is a set of clearly differentiated mechanisms involved in the irradiation process which correspond to those discussed in the interaction process with transparent materials.

First, the beam that is applied has a Gaussian intensity distribution. This implies that there are central areas where the beam irradiation intensity is much higher at the edges (Fig. 1.4).

Also, the size of the Gaussian beam is determined by its "waist", which varied in size when propagated in a way that its value, in the smaller area is given by W_0. This value is measured when the intensity of the distribution of Gaussian decreases to $1/e^2$ of the maximum value in the central area. It is essential to perform the W0 measurements correctly for two reasons. In the first place it determines the value of the intensity when it is irradiating per unit area and therefore with the mechanism involved in the tissue breakdown, and in the second place because it determines the time of irradiation of the area where the sample moves at a given speed to perform a cut, so the Fluence parameter depends indirectly on it.[14-16,22]

To calculate the energy density during laser-induced optical breakdown (LIOB), the focal diameter must be determined by the knife-edge method that is a beam-profiling optical method that gives accurate precision of the cross-sectioned laser beam parameters.

When we have moderate numerical aperture (NA), the spatial distribution of the deposited energy is influenced by non-linear process of self-focusing and plasma defocusing that leads to the filamentation and streak formation in the tissue. For the case of water and glass it has been found that NA ≥ 0.9 is necessary.[12]

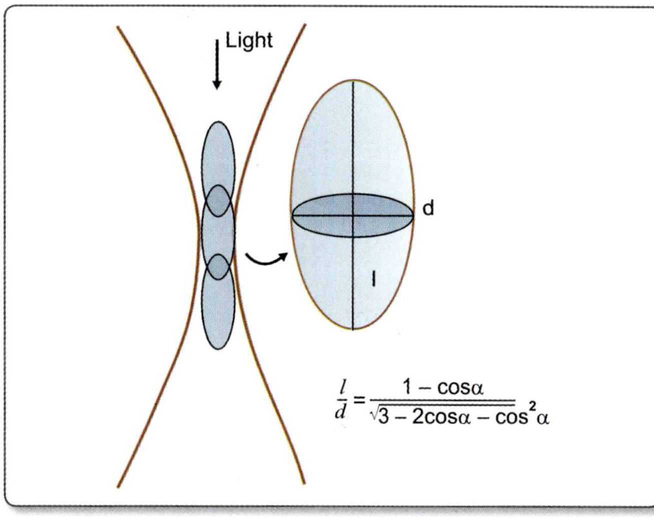

Fig. 1.4: Representing the targeted area of a Gaussian beam. We amplified, in 3D, the smallest area. The equation that allows us to mathematically calculate this area has also been included. α represents the angle given by the NA of the microscope's lens used for the focusing[12,14]

Figure 1.5 presents the principal of this method and the experimental results for a long working objective 10X with NA = 0.3, and with a wavelength of 800 nm.

The evolution of the width W_0 is approximated by the following beam waist function:

$$W_Z = W_0\sqrt{1+\left(\frac{\lambda z}{\pi W_0^2}\right)^2}$$

The shape distribution of the irradiance within the focal volume is important in order to know the distribution of free-electrons produced during the optical breakdown. This volume can be approximated by an ellipsoid with short

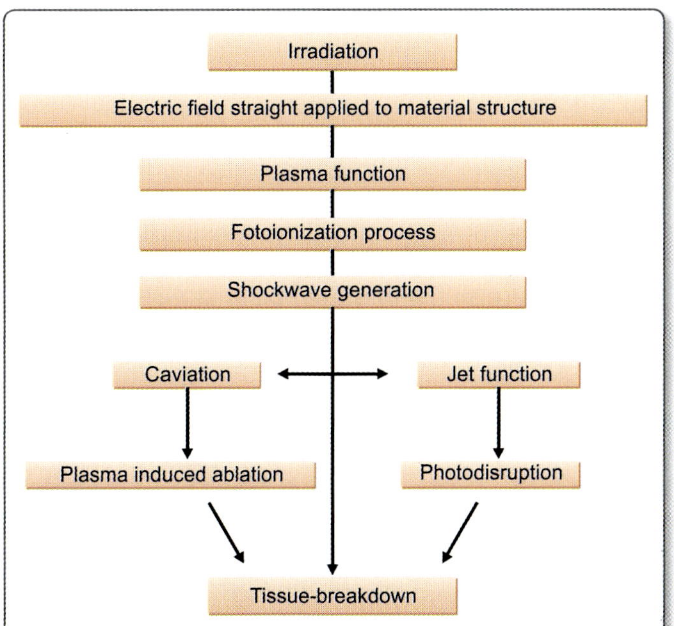

Fig. 1.3: Mechanisms occurring during the irradiation process[3]

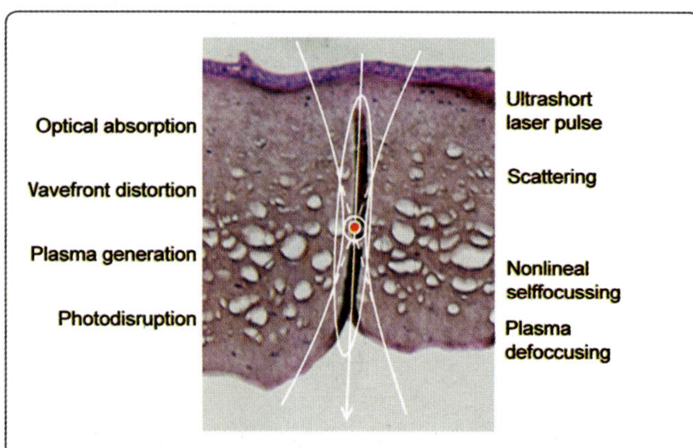

Fig. 1.5: Physical processes involved in the propagation of an ultrashort laser pulse into corneal tissue

axis "d" and long axis "l". The short axis "d" is given by the diameter of the central maximum of the airy pattern in the focal plane and is given by:

$$d = 1.22 \frac{\lambda}{NA}$$

Where λ is the vacuum wavelength of the light and "l" is given by the relation:

$$\frac{l}{d} = \frac{1 - \cos\alpha}{\sqrt{3 - 2\cos\alpha - \cos^2\alpha}}$$

Where α is the angle of numerical aperture for very large solid angles. If λ = 800 nm and NA = 1.3 then d = 0.75 µm and l = 1.8 µm (Fig. 1.5).[3,13,15]

Similarly, the W_0 variation along the focusing area depends on the wavelength and the numerical aperture of the optical system used for focusing. All these parameters and their definitions and the calculation of their numerical values are given in Appendix.

Laser-induced optical breakdown (Fig. 1.4) plays a significant role in the mechanism of plasma-mediated photodisruption, the most important interaction between femtosecond pulses and tissues. LIOB requires a small focal spot size to achieve the threshold Fluence (energy/area) for plasma formation.[3] For example, in same experiments, because the main component in the human corneal tissue is water (approximately 75%), the threshold is to 2.0 J/cm^2 in the case of pulses with 350 fs duration.

One important point of laser-tissue interaction is that the Fluence threshold for optical breakdown decreases with the pulse duration, resulting in a reduction in pulse energy, shock-wave range and cavitation bubble size.

Moreover, during the propagation of light inside the tissue absorption and scattering effects reproduced which significantly decrease the intensity of the beam. Plasma is generated in the area of optical breakdown as well as a clear distortion of the beam and the auto-focalization effect previously mentioned. Finally, we can see the creating of bubbles and a certain blur due to the action of the plasma. The energy transferred to the shockwave is between 1–5% of the incidence. The generation of the effect of vaporization and the expansion of the irradiated area need between 15–25% of energy, and finally, the production of plasma between 70–90%. Clearly, this energy mix is an approximation, but still it highlights the importance of the focalization systems that are used.[3]

As we have comment the spatial resolution of femtosecond laser surgery is determined by the width of the free-electron distribution that is the function of focalized size and peak intensity. For a high numerical aperture the focal volume has an elipsoid form. However, we can consider it to be a spherical shape in a first approximation, for evaluation of thermal diffusion time "td" that is given approximately by:

$$td = \frac{d^2}{2K}$$

Where K is the thermal diffusivity and d the focal diameter, if we like to have thermal confinement, the laser exposure is much shorter than the thermal diffusion time.[3,12]

With the multiphoton ionization process, the half-width of free-electron distribution of 0.19 µm for λ = 800 nm and NA = 1.3, but the half-width of temperature distribution is 0.39 µm and 0.73 µm, resulting from irradiation with a pulse duration of 10 µm and 10 ms, respectively.

At 80 MHz repetition rate the dissection is possible to perform in low-density plasma regime at nJ energies below the optical breakdown threshold. In Figure 1.6, we present the intratissue thermic action produced in a chicken cornea irradiated with a 76 MHz repetition rate. The second effect in this process is the shrinkage of tissue.

The pulse duration is another essential parameter used. As shown in Figure 1.3, commercial systems use pulses of 200–800 fs, which permits the use of high peak intensities which are very energetic, given that the repetition rates are range in kHz.[9]

We must remember that the temporal pulse size increases as it propagates through the different elements of the optical system and we should, at all times, refer to the temporal size of the irradiation area.

An easy way to measure the width of the pulse is by spectral width in nanometers (nm) of the irradiation beam. Pulse widths of a 4 nm spectral lead us to times of 500 fs.

The fact that the tissue structure has a regular shape is also of great importance as it allows us to control the losses produced by scattering.

In recent years, there has been ex vivo studies designed to use lasers focused on 800 nm with high repetition frequencies of 76–80 MHz and pulse energies near nJ.[13,17,21]

The aim of these studies is to reduce as far as possible the side effects on the irradiated areas as well as to avoid possible damage to the retina due to the propagation of the beam which does not interact with the tissue. Figure 1.6 shows some results of the experiments conducted in this field.

Köning[20] works with an 80 MHz repetition rate, 800 nm wavelength and pulse duration of 170 fs. The size of the photodisruption area is 1 µm and has irradiated with an optical objective 40X (NA = 1.3). He obtained excellent results in flap production. On the other hand, Gualda[11,17] worked with a 1 MHz repetition rate, 120 fs and a pulse energy of 1.7 µJ with a 20X objective (NA = 0.4). In this

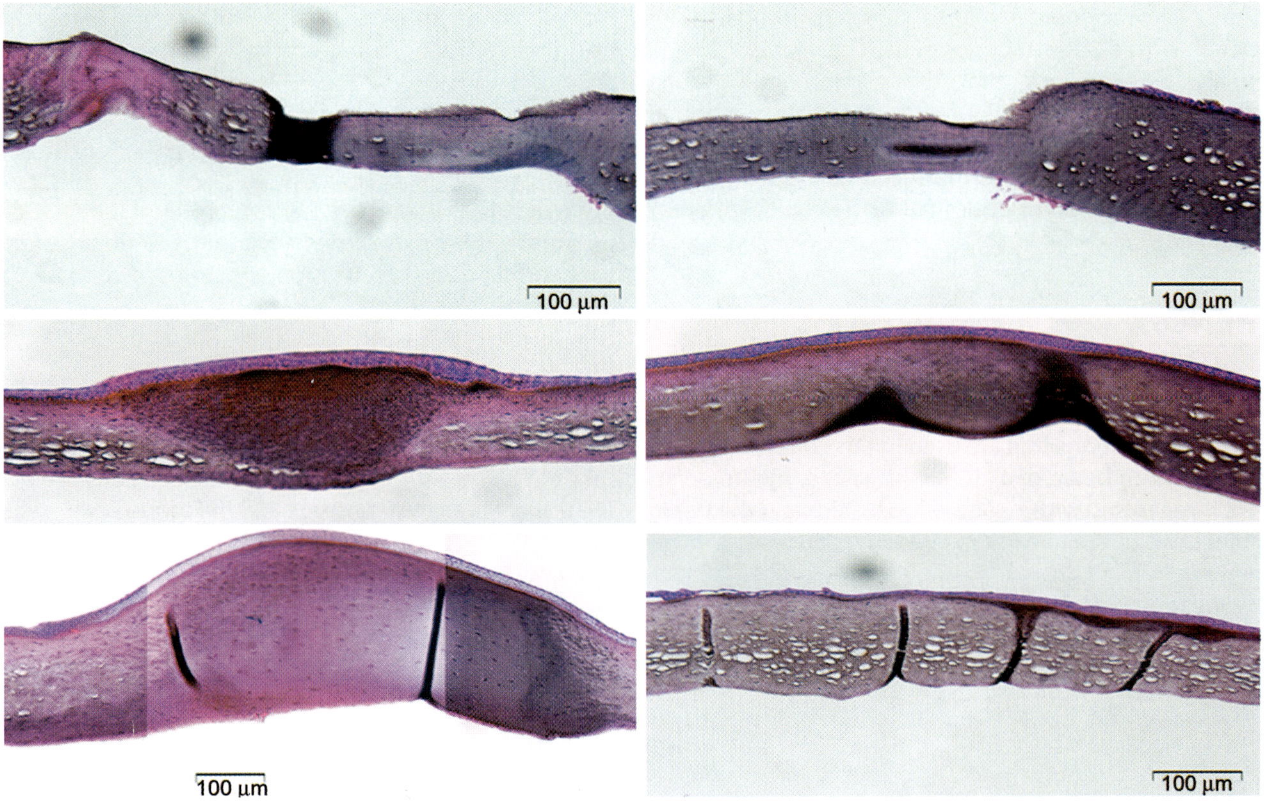

Fig. 1.6: Internal thermic action in corneal tissue (chicken) due to laser irradiation with high repetition rate frequency

paper, intrastromal photodisruption has been observed with multiphoton microscopy.

Recent techniques have proposed intratissue refractive index shaping (IRIS), creating periodic structures in the corneal stroma to change the refractive index. Huxlin proposed this method as an alternative method for refractive surgery.[10,16] Hovhannisyah[18,19] proposed a photo-modification collagen structure with a laser of 80 MHz repetition frequency, with a wavelength centered in the 780 nm, pulse duration of 120 fs and the intensity was between 10–50 mW, irradiated with a 20X objective (NA = 0.5).

All these studies give us information about the experimental evidence regarding the photodisruption process or photomodification of the corneal intrastromal with a high number of pulses per second and low energy pulses.

As an example of this interaction, Figure 1.6 shows the image of a histological section of a cornea of a chicken irradiated with a fs laser with a duration of 170 fs and a repetition rate of 76 MHz, and 800 nm wavelength. This result has been deliberately chosen to demonstrate the different effects that occur during the irradiation of this kind and have been discussed in this chapter.

FUTURE DIRECTIONS

As previously mentioned, this is a technology that is currently being developed and a lot has to be learnt and developed, but is tremendously potential in corneal surgery.[23,24]

On the other hand, there is the proposal discussed before regarding the study with high repetition lasers and pulse energies near to nanojoules, aiming to improve and optimize a clearer reduction of the side effects. Furthermore, we have the possibility to use the lasers with longer wavelengths than that used at this moment where tissue penetration is greater, although there may be scattering problems.[9]

Finally, we say that some of the improvement is due to the use of new technologies. Lasers that are more compact, smaller in size, lower in price and are optically compatible with ablation technologies that use ultraviolet lasers.[9]

Recently, we have increased the field of development that has been proposed lately to study the processes of interaction with tissue structures of the crystalline.

Finally, we conclude that the experimental results analyzed in recent bibliographies suggest optimal pulse duration for a corneal photodisruption and with a shorter femtosecond duration range with high repetition frequency and irradiation optics compatible with different wavelengths.

APPENDIX

This appendix provides some information about the important parameters that we need for the Fluence and dosimetry calculations that we used in this chapter.

The Gaussian beam of a laser, in specified, by the beam waist. It is measured with a knife-edge system and the beam diameter is when the maximum intensity reduces to a value of $1/e^2$, that is, to 13.4%.

The relation between the central-beam intensity (I_0) and the Fluence (F) can be calculated by:

$$I_0 = \frac{P}{\pi\omega^2_{\frac{1}{e}}}$$

$$F = \frac{Q}{\pi\omega^2_{\frac{1}{e}}}$$

Where P is the radiant power in Watts (W) and Q is the radian energy in Joules (J).

If the beam radius is specified at the $1/e^2$ of maximum intensity, then we must apply:

$$\omega_{\frac{1}{e}} \cong 0.707\omega_{\frac{1}{e^2}}$$

The intensity distribution of a Gaussian beam, I (f, z), is:

$$I(f,z) = \left(\frac{\omega_0}{\omega(z)}\right)^2 \times e^{\frac{2f^2}{\omega^2(z)}}$$

Where $f = \sqrt{x^2 + y^2}$ is the radial distance and Z is the axial distance from the beam waist.

When an ultrashort laser pulse travels through the elements of an objective microscope, the pulses are subject to temporal broadening due to group-velocity distortion. The pulse in this case is referred to as a "chirped pulsed."

Using the dispersion parameter, the length of the optical material, the chirp C of the pulse associated with the time-beam width is given by:

$$\zeta A\omega = 4\ln(2)\sqrt{1+c^2}$$

We can evaluate the pulse length, τ, at the output of the material, if we know the pulse incident in the material τ_0, using the following equation:

$$\zeta = \zeta_0 \sqrt{\left[1 + \frac{4\ln(2)\beta_2 ZC}{\zeta_0^2}\right]^2 + \left[\frac{4\ln(2)\beta_2 Z}{\zeta_0^2}\right]^2}$$

Where β_2 is the dispersion parameter of materials.

Finally, it is possible to calculate the time pulse width if we can measure the emission spectrum of the laser using the following equation:

$$\zeta = 0.441\frac{\lambda_0^2}{c\Delta\lambda}$$

Where λ_0 is the central wavelength, $\Delta\lambda$ is the spectral FWHM, and we suppose that we have a transform-limited chirp-free Gaussian pulse (c = 300 nm/fs).

ACKNOWLEDGMENTS

This study has been supported in part by a grant from the Spanish Ministry of Science and Innovation, Centro para el Desarrollo Tecnológico Industrial (CDTI), CENIT: "Customized Eye Care", CeyeC (CEN-20091021).

REFERENCES

1. Roach WP, Thompson ET. Selected papers on Ultrashort laser pulse bioeffects. SPIE Milestone Series. 2002;174.
2. Krasnov MM. Q-Switched laser goniopuncture. Arch Ophthalmol. 1974;92(1):37-41.
3. Niemz, MH. Laser-tissue interactions. Fundamentals and applications. Third, revised Edition. Biological and medical physics, biomedical engineering. Springer. 2003.
4. Prasad PN. Introduction to Biophotonics. Wiley-Interscience. Jonh Wiley and Sons. 2003.
5. Juhasz T, Loesel FH, Kurtz RM, Horvath C, Bille JF, Mourou, G. Corneal refractive surgery with femtosecond lasers. IEEE Journal of Selected Topics in Quantum Electronics. 1999;4(5):902-10.
6. Loesel FH, Niemz MH, Bille JF, Juhasz T. Laser-induced optical breakdown on hard and soft tissues and its dependence on the pulse duration: experiment and model. IEEE Journal of Quantum Electronics. 1996;10(32):1717-22.
7. Tien A, Backus S, Kapteyn H, Murnane M, Mourou G. Short-pulse laser damage in transparent materials as a function of pulse duration. Phys Rev Lett. 1999;82:3883-6.
8. Schaffer C, Brodeur A, Mazur, E. Laser-induced breakdown and damage in bulk transparent materials induced by tightly focused femtosecond laser pulses. Meas Sci Technol. 2001;12:1784.
9. Plamann K, Aptel F, Arnold C L, Courjaud A, Crotti C, Deloison F, et al. Ultrashort pulse laser surgery of the cornea and the sclera. Journal of Optics. 2010;12(8):DOI: 084002.

10. Ding L, Knox WH, Bühren J, Nagy LJ, Huxlin KR. Intratissue refractive index shaping (IRIS) of the cornea and lens using a low-pulse-energy femtosecond laser oscillator. Invest Ophthalmol Vis Sci. 2008;49(12):5332-9.
11. Mao SS, Quéré F, Guizard S, Mao X, Russo RE, Petite G, Martin P. Dynamics of femtosecond laser interactions with dielectrics. Applied Physics A Materials Science and Processing. 2004;7(79):1695-709.
12. Vogel A, Noack J, Hüttman G, Paltauf G. Mechanisms of femtosecond laser nanosurgery of cells and tissues. Applied Physics B. 2005;8(81):1015-47.
13. Zhou J, Chen JK, Zhang Y. Numerical modeling of transient progression of plasma formation in biological tissues induced by short laser pulses. Applied Physics B. 2008;90(1):141-8.
14. Grill S, Stelzer EHK. Method to calculate lateral and axial gain factors of optical setups with a large solid angle. JOSA A. 1999;16(11):2658-65.
15. Netz R, Feurer T, Wolleschensky R, Sauerbrey R. Measurement of the pulse-front distortion in high-numerical-aperture optics. Applied Physics B Lasers and Optics. 2000;6(70):833-7.
16. Nagy LJ, Ding L, Xu L, Knox WH, Huxlin KR. Potentiation of femtosecond laser intratissue refractive index shaping (IRIS) in the living cornea with sodium fluorescein. Invest Ophthalmol Vis Sci. 2010;51(2):850-6.
17. Gualda EJ, Vázquez de Aldana JR, Martínez-García MC, Moreno P, Hernández-Toro J, Roso L, et al. Femtosecond infrared intrastromal ablation and backscattering-mode adaptive-optics multiphoton microscopy in chicken corneas. Biomed Opt Express. 2011;2(11):2950-60.
18. Hovhannisyan V, Ghazaryan A, Chen YF, Chen SJ, Dong CY. Photophysical mechanisms of collagen modification by 80 MHz femtosecond laser. Opt Express. 2010;18(23):24037-47.
19. Hovhannisyan V, Lo W, Hu C, Chen SJ, Dong CY. Dynamics of femtosecond laser photo-modification of collagen fibers. Opt Express. 2008;16(11):7958-68.
20. König K, Krauss O, Riemann I. Intratissue surgery with 80 MHz nanojoule femtosecond laser pulses in the near infrared. Opt Express. 2002;10(3):171-6.
21. Hoffart L, Lassonde P, Légaré F, Vidal F, Sanner N, Utéza O, et al. Surface ablation of corneal stroma with few-cycle laser pulses at 800 nm. Opt Express. 2011;19(1):230-40.
22. Nuzzo V, Savoldelli M, Legeais JM, Plamann K. Self-focusing and spherical aberrations in corneal tissue during photodisruption by femtosecond laser. J Biomed Opt. 2010;15(3):DOI:038003.
23. Han M, Giese G, Zickler L, Sun H, Bille J. Mini-invasive corneal surgery and imaging with femtosecond lasers. Opt Express. 2004;12(18):4275-81.
24. Tse C, Zohdy MJ, Ye JY, O'Donnell M. Penetration and precision of subsurface photodisruption in porcine skin tissue with infrared femtosecond laser pulses. IEEE Trans Biomed Engineering. 2008;55:1211-8.

Chapter

2 Femtosecond Laser Technology for Ophthalmic Surgeons and Clinicians: Understanding a New Emerging Technology

Felipe Soria, Jorge L Alió

CHAPTER OUTLINE

Understanding the basics of a laser energy system:
- Energy levels in the atom
- Principles of atomic stimulation for the generation of energy in a laser system:
  - Pumping and inversion population
  - Principles of emission radiation

The use of lasers in ophthalmology: variables involved:
- Electromagnetic spectrum
- Wavelength
- Frequency
- Relation between energy and wavelength
- Relation between energy and time
- Numerical aperture
- Speed repetition rates: total time procedure and total energy delivered to the cornea
- Corneal femtosecond laser vs cataract femtosecond laser

Laser-tissue interaction with a femtosecond laser system:
- Femtosecond laser beam output
  - Pulse anatomy
  - Settings of femtosecond laser

  Stepping on the foot pedal: What it happens in an ocular tissue?
- Creating optical breakdown (photoionization) and plasma formation
- Photodisruption in order to achieve tissue ablation

"Everything should be made as simple as possible, but not simpler."

—**Albert Einstein**

INTRODUCTION

The main goals in every kind of surgery is trying to achieve the maximum effect with the minimal tissue damage possible, accomplishing a painless procedure with a fast recovery and a minimal potential of complications. Unprecedented versatility and huge potential has brought femtosecond laser technology to the cutting edge of this goal in ophthalmic surgery. Our aim in this chapter is to offer to ophthalmic surgeons and clinicians a simplified perspective on the physics involved in the use of femtosecond laser procedures.

In the following text, we present from the beginning the principles of how a laser beam is created and a follow up of all the whole process until the tissue dissection is achieved. In this way, our main interest has been that the reader will have a logical and reasoned step by step of the whole process, thus we believe that the association between concepts that generally the ophthalmologists do not handle, will become clearer.

The text often presents basic issues and is because our purpose is heading to all ophthalmologists and try to bring them to this technology that we are sure is becoming an important part of the present and will be even more in the future in ophthalmology.

What is written in the next lines are behaviors of the matter inside the atom, so the reader has to understand with imagination that this are subatomic concepts of time, energy, pressure and speed. We have made provision of images because we believe that always an image is worth one thousand words.

This chapter has the only goal to provide ophthalmologists a simple (but no simpler) way of understanding how this technology interacts with matter. It is a chapter hosted from ophthalmologists to be understood by other ophthalmologists.

BASIC CONCEPTS: CREATING LIGHT AMPLIFICATION STIMULATED EMISSION RADIATION

Energy Levels

The nucleus of an atom of every material is surrounded by a cloud of electrons that is formed by the alternation movements of the electrons from different orbits (Fig. 2.1). Such "jumping" process to an upper orbit or to a lower orbit requires the absorption or the emission of energy respectively in terms of a photon. This is the concept of energy levels[1] (Fig. 2.1).

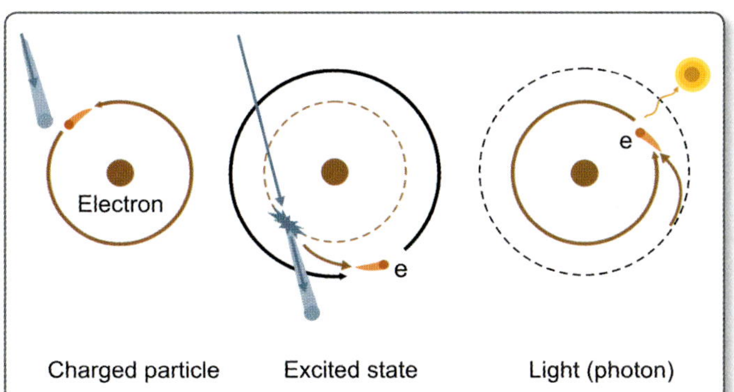

Fig. 2.1: Absorption of energy makes the electron to "jump" to an upper level of energy and become an excited state. A decrease in energy level will result in an emission of light

In ophthalmology femtosecond laser systems, one of the most common material used is Neodymium (Nd), a rare earth doped media. In one atom of Nd we find 60 electrons that are alternating in the 6 levels of energy (Fig. 2.2). In the following paragraphs we will explain how the electrons move from one level to another and why it is beneficial for a laser system to have 6 levels of energy.

Normal Population, Pumping and Inversion Population: Stimulation

In the configuration described previously of our atom of Nd that has 60 electrons and 6 energy levels, the normal population of electrons behavior if it is not stimulated by an external photon (laser in off position), the majority of the 60 electrons will be in the ground level (level 0), in other words, they are not charged with a photon.

To have an efficient laser system we need to compel the majority of electrons in upper levels. We remember that electron population that is in upper levels will provide of more photons to the laser system.

In a process called pumping, an external diode laser is focused inside the Nd:glass gain media. This laser beam will pump millions of photons to stimulate each of the 60 electrons of the millions of atoms of Nd. The majority of the electrons that were in the ground level will absorb this stimulus and will climb to the upper levels. Changing the localization of the majority of the electrons from the ground level to upper levels is called population inversion.

An important thing to take in account and we will mention it later, is that when we select the amount of energy that we want to use in our treatment, what we are doing is pumping more photons with the diode laser to the

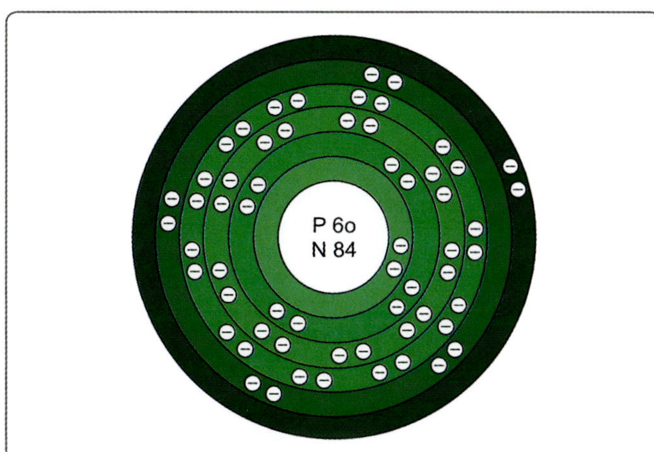

Fig. 2.2: Electron configuration of neodymium (Nd)

Nd:glass system so more electrons of Nd are stimulated and more energy can be assessed.

What Goes Up, Must Come Down and Out (Emission Radiation)

Gaining energy has allowed electrons to "climb" to upper levels and achieve population inversion. The electrons must come down in a certain moment in order to release the photons they have gained in a process called emission. The two ways for them to emit this radiation (photon) are spontaneously or by receiving an external photon. Having more energy levels provides the system of electrons in different levels that drop down to the subsequent level emitting a photon and still having more energy to emit. For example, one electron that received the necessary energy to climb to position 6 will drop to energy level 5 emitting a photon, but still has 4 energy levels to continue descending and emitting photons in each descend. If we contrast this situation with only a one energy level, the electron will receive energy to climb to the only upper level and when it descend, will only have the opportunity to emit only one time before returning to the ground level (Fig. 2.3).

Immediately the electron; (a) emits a photon when descending, this photon will impact another electron (b) and will make it also descend, but at the same time it will emit another photon. This process occurs in millions of electrons in the different energy levels, but all of these photons have the same energy component. The tremendous number of photons that are been emitted are moving back and forth between two mirrors and traveling in different frequencies, these different frequencies will interact with each other and in an adding and subtracting natural process (mathematically proved see reference for more information) only one frequency will be achieved. After that, a modelock instrument, will lock the frequency and will convert it to an ultrashort pulse (femtosecond).

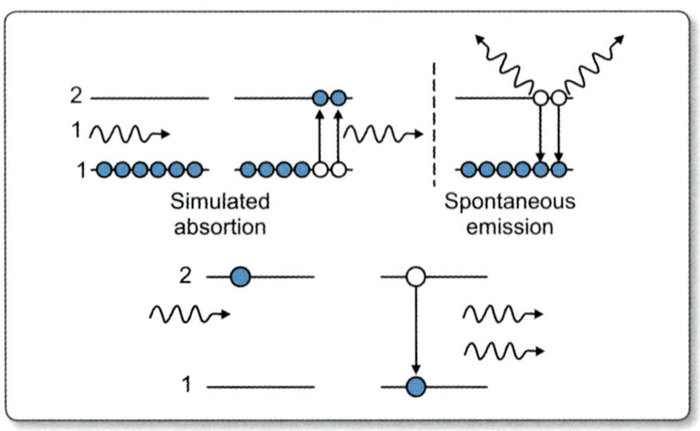

Fig. 2.3: Energy level transition

The laser beam comes out through an out coupling mirror converted in a monochromatic (unique wavelength of 1043 nm), coherent (all photons waves are correlated in space and time) type of light.[2]

WAVES IN TIME AND SPACE: UNDERSTANDING LASERS IN OPHTHALMOLOGY

Electromagnetic Spectrum

It is not the interest of this chapter to explain the complete electromagnetic spectrum, but it is necessary to explain the basic principle properties of the waves to understand how they travel in time and space.

Wavelength

The distance between two points on a wave, which have the same value and the same rate of change of the value of a parameter (Fig. 2.4).[1]

Frequency

The number of times that a periodic function or vibration repeats itself in a specified time.

Lasers in ophthalmology range from the far infrared wavelength 10,600 μm to the ultraviolet wavelength of 193 μm.

The statement above is determined by Planck´s constant that indicates the energy in one photon of electromagnetic radiation to the frequency of that radiation ($h = 6.626176 \times 10^{-34}$ joule-seconds).

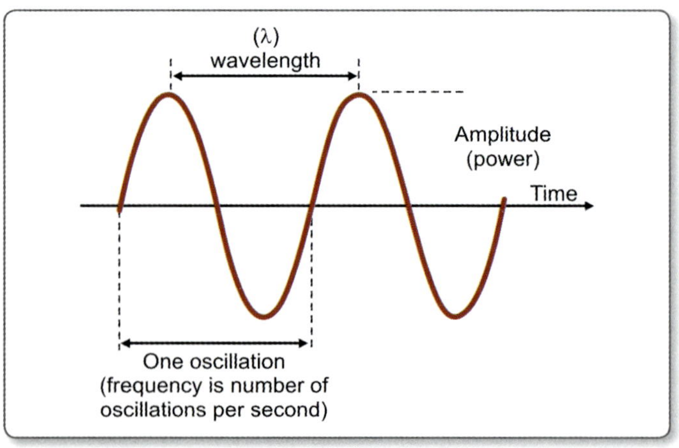

Fig. 2.4: Wave anatomy

Relation between Energy and Wavelength

The energy of the photon is determined by:

$$E = hc/\lambda$$

E = energy
h (Planck´s constant) = 6.626176 × 10^{-34} joule-seconds
c (speed of light) = 3 × 10º8
λ = wavelength
Examples:
How much energy is carried out by a single photon with a wavelength of 1,030 µm (femtosecond)?

E = (6.626176 × 10^{-34} J-s × 3 × 10º8 m/s)/1,03 × 10º-6m

E= 0.00000000000000000019299541747572982 J

How much energy is carried out by a single photon with a wavelength of 193 µm (Excimer)?

E = (6.626176 × 10^{-34} J-s × 3 × 10º8 m/s)/193 × 10º-6m

E = 0.000000000000000000001029975544041 5 J

As we can observe in the examples above and in Table 2.1,[4] if the wavelength is increased, the amount of energy in a photon decreases. The amount of energy will define the type of interaction with the matter, although it is not determinant. Another important variable that will delimit the laser-matter interaction is time.

Relation between Energy and Time

The Nd:YAG (neodymium-doped yttrium aluminum garnet) works almost in the same wavelength that our Nd:glass, but it has a pulse duration of nanoseconds instead of femtoseconds. So why do we use a femtosecond laser if both produce photodisruption? The main concept that summarizes all is to achieve the maximum energy possible according to the wavelength in the shortest time possible in order to accomplish photodisruption with the minimal collateral damages.[5]

In the following formula, the anterior statement is explained in a simple way.

Power (W) = Energy (mJ)/Time

We can deduce that decreasing the time of the laser pulse (time of interaction with the matter) we can achieve more power at a constant energy determined by the wavelength.

In a practical point of view:

When doing a YAG laser procedure, we can manage the energy (mJ), this setting allow us to accomplish the photodisruption of the posterior capsule with more less 4 mJ with a pulse duration of 10 nanosecond.[6] In a femtosecond procedure with less energy of 0.45–0.8 mJ[6-8] we can also achieve photodisruption by reducing the pulse duration to less than 500 femtoseconds (fs).

The side effect of greater energy is disruption of the surrounding tissue and this is what we have to avoid. It is estimated that the tissue damage of the nanosecond laser is of 100 µm[9] in comparison with the 1µm of the fs.

With the variables explained above (wavelength, energy, pulse duration and power), the laser beam interacting with the matter will achieve photodisruption with the minimal collateral damages. To achieve extreme precision one more variable is needed.

Extreme Precision: Numerical Aperture

One of the most important and critical components in a laser system is the beam delivery device. Numerical aperture (NA) is defined as the sine of the angle of the marginal ray coming from the focal point, multiplied by the refractive index of the medium from which the input beam comes. The optics present in the mechanism is an amazing technology and the NA of the objective will determine the spot size, hence the extreme precision. The spot size will contain all the energy in a diameter greater than 1µm.
The following equation explains the importance of the NA:

NA = w/f
NA = Numerical Aperture
W = Power
f = focal distance

Table 2.1: Comparison of different lasers used in ophthalmology

Laser	*Wavelength*	*Energy (eV)*	*Electromagnetic spectrum*	*Effect in tissue*
Carbon Dioxide	10,600 µm	0.138	Far infrared	Photothermal
Nd:YAG	1,064 µm	1.16	Near infrared	Photodisruption
Femtosecond	1,030–1,060 µm	3.49–4.66	Near infrared	Plasma-mediated ablation/photodisruption
Krypton	647–531 µm	2.3	Visible light	Photochemical (Coagulation)
Argon	514–488 µm	2.5	Visible light	Photochemical (Coagulation)
Yellow	561 µm	2.20		Photochemical (Coagulation)
Excimer	193 µm	6.4	Far Ultraviolet	Photochemical (Coagulation)

Achieving the larger NA possible the energy delivered will condense in a decreased spot size. This allows to use smaller pulse energies.[4]

The two ways to increase the NA are to increase the lens diameter and the other, is to decrease the focal distance as seen in the Figure 2.5.

Speed Repetition Rates: Total Time Procedure and Total Energy Delivered to the Cornea

Hertz is defined as how many cycles are produced in 1 second. The first corneal femtolaser system to get the 510 K clearance for creating Laser-Assisted in Situ Keratomileusis (LASIK) flaps worked in the order of the 6 kHz and the time it took to complete a 9.0 mm flap was of 1 minute.[10] Now days, most corneal femtolaser systems work in an average between 60 to 150 kHz, this means 60.000 to 150.000 cycles per second, a 9.0 mm lasik flap procedure is completed in less than 20 seconds.[3,8,9]

Only one femtolaser machine works in the MHz, it is not published the exact speed pulse repetition, but it is at least 1.000.000 cycles per second. Although increasing the speed pulse rate does not mean that, the procedure will be timeless.

Low repetition rates (kHz) lasers work with high pulse energy (mJ), meanwhile the laser that uses high repetition rates (MHz) do this with low pulse energy (nJ) (Fig. 2.6). Clinically there is no difference in the tissue dissection, but surgeons need to understand that in low repetition rates, the space between each spot is increased and this can result in uncut areas or bridges of tissue. The spacing can be managed by the user. In high repetition rates (MHz), the energy used is less (nanojoules vs microjoules), but the total energy disposed in the cornea is bigger because of the increased amount of spots. Total energy disposed to the cornea finally is important. One of the benefits of decreasing energy is to decrease the potential for transient light-sensitivity syndrome.[11]

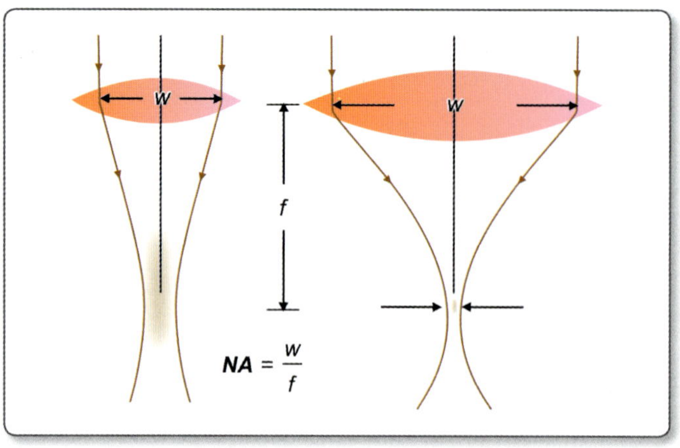

Fig. 2.5: Numerical aperture concept

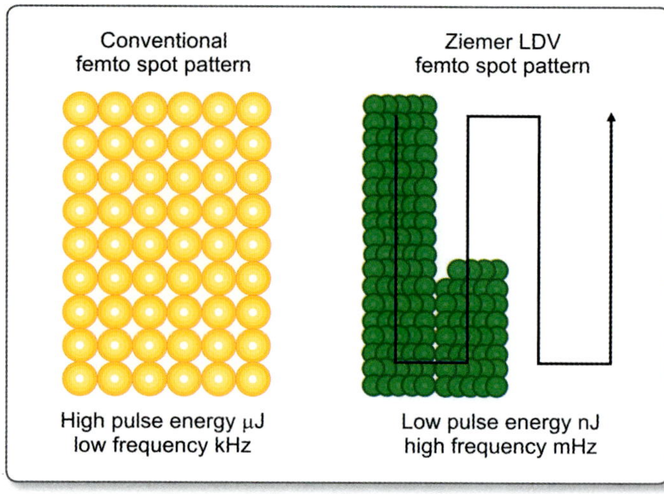

Fig. 2.6: Femtosecond lasers: Low frequency rates (kHz) versus high frequency rates (mHz)

Corneal Femtosecond Laser vs Cataract Femtosecond Laser

Performing photodisruption in approximately 8 mm from the corneal surface is the main difference between a femtosecond laser system for cornea surgery than for cataract surgery. The different anatomy found in patients makes necessary that femto laser cataract systems be provided with optical coherence tomography technology in order to assure the maximum precision.

In addition of this depth difference, higher laser power is needed to reach the nucleus fragmentation considering in this concept the type of cataract. Like it was explained above, the pumping process and specific laser materials are involved to increase the laser power.

Another important issue comparing both laser systems is that in femtosecond lasers for cataract the NA must be smaller; this is because the cone angle beam is limited by the iris. Decreasing the NA will increase our spot size and will also allow a major energy.

Hopefully, in the next months we can be able to use a unique laser system to perform more than 20 ophthalmic procedures that have been proposed.[3]

LASER-MATTER INTERACTION

Femtosecond Laser Beam Output

Pulse Anatomy

In order to understand how the laser interacts with the matter, we must first take a look to the anatomy of the laser beam output. In the following figure we show the characteristics of the femtosecond laser beam.

Settings of Femtosecond Laser[9]

a. Fixed Settings
   - Laser spot size: < 3 µm (characterization, binder)
   - Speed pulse repetition rate: 60 kHz or 150 kHz (60.000 times per second or 150.000 times per second)
   - Pulse duration: 600–800 fs
   - Raster Energy: 0.45 to 0.8 microjoules/pulse (Total per procedure: 1.3 J)
   - Wavelength: 1053

b. Variable Settings
   - Mean pulse energy: 100 mW
   - Distance between laser pulses

Stepping on the Foot Pedal

Immediately when you turn on your femtosecond laser machine, the electricity will activate the diode laser starting the pumping in order to produce the population inversion in the warm up process. The laser beam created will be reflected in a series of complex moving mirrors that are controlled by precise electrical motors. These mirrors allow the movement in the horizontal plane of the beam, meanwhile the optics situated at the end of the path of the laser beam will manage to control the vertical component (deepness of the focus).

Pressing the foot pedal will initiate the tissue ablation by firstly opening the shutter and letting the laser beam out. The objective of the laser beam is to achieve an optical breakdown of the matter, thus to achieve this characteristics of the beam are it´s wavelength (1053 nm), the ultrashort period of pulse time (800 fs) and the tightly focused laser beam (>1 µm) into the tissue by a high numerical objective.[12]

Achieving optical breakdown will produce two different concepts that have in common the tissue ablation. The first one called plasma-induced ablation determines a physics process and the second one is called photodisruption and describes a mechanical behavior of matter.

A Matter of Exciting Electrons: Creating Optical Breakdown (Photoionization) and Plasma Formation[12,13]

Like we all know if we apply a large amount of heat to an ice cube (a solid), it soon will go through different states of matter transforming the atoms into liquid and gas. If we had more energy, we could convert the gas into plasma. Plasma is called the 4th matter and is still not totally understood by physicists. Regards this, in our specialty we can understand how plasma can make the dissection in the cornea.

Matter has free electrons, and the human cornea, the anterior capsule, the lens and the whole eye are not the exception. Free electrons are not orbiting the atom but are attached to it in the form of static electricity. As we know, an atom has a neutral charge (same amount of electrons and protons), releasing only one electron (in this case a free electron) will determine that the atom will be positive ionized. Achieving ionization by a photon (laser beam) is what is called photoionization or optical breakdown. In other words, when ionizing radiation impinges on matter, large quantities of free electrons are released, thus releasing a 800 fs pulse, with an energy disposed of 0.45 to 0.8 microjoules will discharge the cornea stroma atoms from the free electrons. Optical breakdown is of extreme importance because it will trigger plasma formation (physical process), photodisruption (mechanical process) and subsequently tissue dissection.

Producing photoionization of one atom, will release one electron, these electron has gain energy and will accelerate (kinetic energy), the accelerated electron will "hit" another electron (of another atom) releasing it, resulting in two free electrons, each of them with less individual kinetic energy that the initial electron (Fig. 2.7). Again and again free electrons of atoms will continue to receive incoming photons and will continue striking other atoms.[13-16] With the increasing electron density at a very high temperature, tissue in the focus point is vaporized and plasma induced ablation is achieved.

A Matter of Bubbles: Photodisruption in Order to Achieve Tissue Ablation

Keeping in mind that the laser beam is focused in the corneal tissue with extreme precision, the high kinetic energy formed by the excitation of the free electrons and the adiabatic rise of temperature will accomplish the formation of a microplasma bubble containing water and carbon dioxide. Hypersonic speed expansion of carbon dioxide inside the microplasma bubble (a size of 0.5 um to several micrometers depending on the beam characteristics) due to high temperature will create shock waves[17,18] that will elongate the surrounding tissue determined by the collagen fibrils. Ultimately will slow down to the speed of sound creating, will lose energy and velocity as it propagates, and when it stops it will dissipate as an acoustic wave. Speed of sound in water, for instance, is 1483 m/s at 37ºC, laser-induced shock waves typically reach speeds of up to 5000 m/s.[16] In addition, the microplasma bubble in formation, with its high levels of kinetic energy in a surrounding like the corneal stroma, where pressure outside the microplasma bubble is high, the kinetic energy is transformed to potential energy, converting these bubble into a cavitational one. The maximum diameter that the cavitation bubble can reach is 10 to100 um. Finally, the cavitation bubble will implode and the water and carbon dioxide are absorbed by endothelial cell pump action.

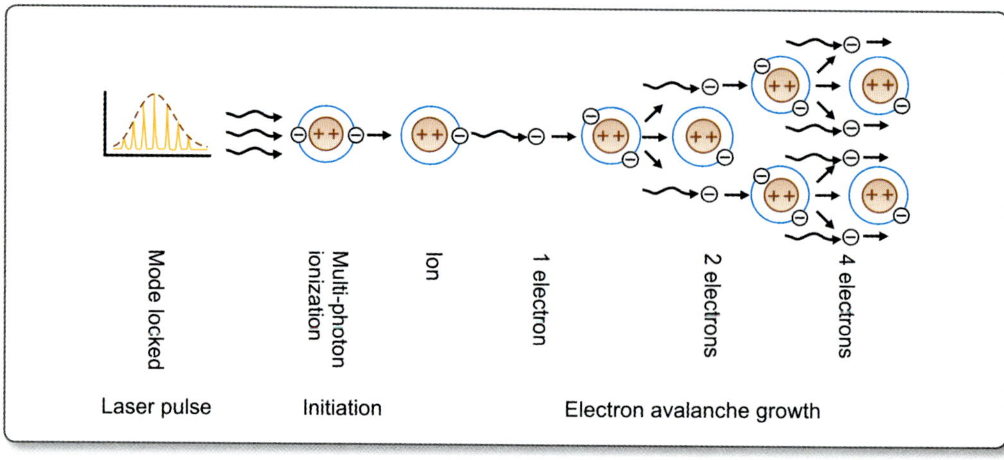

Fig. 2.7: Electron avalanche

The reduced shock wave and cavitation bubble effects of the femtosecond laser result in more localized tissue damage. Therefore, a more confined surgical effect should be expected from a femtosecond laser than that from picosecond (or nanosecond) lasers. This indicates a potential benefit from the applications of femtosecond laser technology to intraocular microsurgery.[19]

Reaching the end, the reader can infer that the electrons have a primary role in the whole process. Electrons are the source of energy in achieving population inversion, creating the Laser beam and also, plasma formation. Ultimately, it's a matter of electrons.

In summary, when turning on the femtolaser machine, the pumping process starts in order to achieve population inversion. Once achieved population inversion, the electrons will start to drop down spontaneously creating an emission (photon) that will continue to stimulate other electrons. Finally adding all this stimuli (photons), a laser beam is created and comes out through an out coupling mirror converted in a monochromatic (unique wavelength of 1043 nm), coherent (all photons waves are correlated in space and time) type of light that will stop in a shutter.

Pressing the pedal will open the shutter and will allow the laser beam to come out through the optics that has a defined NA. The laser beam has a defined laser spot size (< 3 µm), a speed pulse repetition rate (60 kHz or 150 kHz), pulse duration (600–800 fs), raster energy (0.45 to 0.8 microjoules/ pulse), wavelength ( ) and a mean pulse energy (100 mW). These laser beam pulse characteristics will make contact with the matter, achieving optical breakdown, a plasma induced ablation and a photodisruption of the matter.

REFERENCES

1. Hecht E. Optica. Addison-Wesley Iberoamericana, 2000.
2. MIT. Feb. 17, 2010. Laser Fundamentals I | MIT Understanding Lasers and Fiberoptics. Retrieved August 16, 2012, from: http://www.youtube.com/watch?v=rgivGZqFcfY
3. Binder PS, Sarayba M, Ignacio T, et al. Characterization of submicrojoule femtosecond laser corneal tissue dissection. J Cataract Refract Surg. 2008;34:146-52.
4. Slade S. Laser Refractive Cataract Surgery, Science, Medicine and Industry. Wayne, USA. Bryn Mawr Communications LLC. 2012.
5. Kaz Soong H, Baptista Malta J. Femtosecond lasers in ophthalmology. Am J Ophthalmol. 2009;147:189-97.
6. Pepose J, Lubatchowski H. Comparing Femtosecond Lasers: An analysis of commercially available platforms for refractive surgery. Cataract and Refract Surg Today. October, 2008.
7. Lubatschowski H. Overview of commercially available femtosecond lasers in refractive surgery. J Refract Surg. 2008;24(1):S102-7.
8. Binder PS. Femtosecond Lasers. Cataract and Refract Surg Today. October, 2008.
9. Stern D, Schoenlein RW, Puliafito CA, et al. Corneal ablation by nanosecond, picosecond, and femtosecond lasers at 532 and 625 nm. Arch Ophthalmol. 1989;107:587-92.
10. Milas SM, Jing Yong Y, Norris TB, Hollman KW, Emelianov SY, O'Donnell M. Acoustic characterization of microbubble dynamics in laser-induced optical breakdown. Ultrasonics, Ferroelectrics and Frequency Control, IEEE Transactions on. 2003;50:517-22.
11. Stonecipher KG, Dishler JG, Ignacio TS, et al. Transient light sensitivity after femtosecond laser flap creation: clinical findings and management. J Cataract Refract Surg. 2006;32:91-4.

12. Lubatschowski H. Laser Microtomy. Optik and Photonik. 2007;2:49-51.
13. Weiss P. Hot flashes, cold cuts: Ultrafast lasers give power tools a new edge. Science News. 2002;162:315-7.
14. Tsai PS, Blinder P, Migliori BJ, et al. Plasma-mediated ablation: an optical tool for submicrometer surgery on neuronal and vascular systems. Curr Opin Biotechnol. 2009;20:90-9.
15. Vogel A, Busch S, Parlitz U. Shock wave emission and cavitation bubble generation by picosecond and nanosecond optical breakdown in water. J Acoust Soc Am. 1996;100:148-65.
16. Niemz, Markolf H. Laser-Tissue Interactions: Fundamentals and Applications, 3rd edition. New York: Springer; 2007.
17. Faktorovich E. Femtodynamics: A Guide to Laser Settings and Procedure Techniques to Optimize Outcomes with Femtosecond Lasers. Slack Inc; 2009.
18. Milas SM. Acoustic Detection of Microbubble Formation Induced By Enhanced Optical Breakdown of Silver/Dendrimer Nanocomposites, Applied Physics Letters. 2003.
19. Juhasz T, Loesel FH, Kurtz RM, et al. Corneal refractive surgery with femtosecond lasers. IEEE J Select Topics Quantum Electron. 1999;5:902-10.

Chapter

3

Femtosecond Laser Corneal Graft Applications with IntraLase Technology

Juan Gabriel Ortíz, Jorge L Alio

CHAPTER OUTLINE

- IntraLase femtosecond laser technology: Applications to corneal surgery
- IntraLase enabled keratoplasty
  - Understanding cutting profiles. Principles of corneal tissue overlapping by selective customized incision profiles
- Surgical protocol
  - Donor
    - Importance of the control of artificial anterior chamber pressure
  - Recipient
    - Benefits of the IntraLase technology interface design
    - Perfect corneal donor-recipient matching with no oversizing necessary
  - Graft manipulation
  - Suturing technique
- Ad-hoc customization for particular and special cases

INTRALASE FEMTOSECOND LASER ACTION ON CORNEAL TISSUE

Corneal surgery has become of the main use of femtosecond laser technology in ophthalmology since the technology was released nearly a decade ago. Femtosecond laser action resides on the creation of extremely precise incisions within corneal tissue by separating lamellar fibers within the stroma (Fig. 3.1).

Femtosecond tissue dissection is explained under the principles of optical breakdown and laser photodisruption. Laser focuses the photon energy beam at a certain computer-controlled depth into the corneal stroma, concentrating enough energy over the threshold level which frees the chemical bonds that lock electrons into the solid material.[1] This process, known as optical breakdown, and transforms the solid area of tissue covered by the photon beam into vapor state, creating a cavitation gas bubble mainly composed of carbon dioxide and water whose size and position can be precisely controlled.

Cavitation bubble size can vary depending on laser per-pulse energy and occupies a greater space volume than previous solid material, which induces a lamellar tissue separation. The femtosecond laser can be then programed to align several millions of cavitation bubbles to create larger tissue separation in order to compose from single incisions to complex corneal grafts (Fig. 3.2).

Therefore, femto incisions are composed of a huge number of overlapped bubbles placed at a certain distance from each other and specific per-pulse energy. This relationship in spot distance and energy, defines a balance between total energy density per area and treatment time which is characteristic of the various femtosecond laser technologies available.

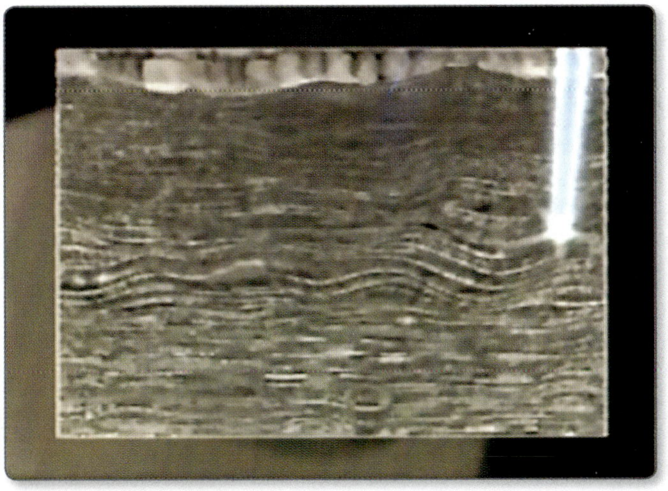

Fig. 3.1: Femtosecond laser pulse energy is focused into the corneal tissue

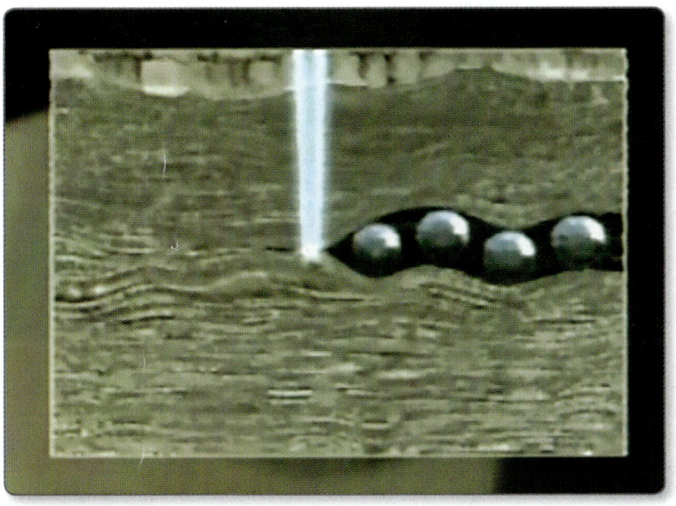

Fig. 3.2: Cavitation bubbles separate stromal lamellas creating a corneal incision

As it is well-known from experienced femtosecond users, this bubble overlap will create micron sized tissue bridges between each bubble felt as velcro effect when mechanically dissection the incisions. Bridges size, number and strength will depend on corneal tissue transparency, laser per-pulse energy, and spot separation. It is then a matter of importance to select the appropriate balance when programing the femtosecond laser to obtain high quality incisions. To optimize incision quality, femtosecond energy pulses need to be then precisely positioned within the corneal tissue to permit bubbles to interact with each other. That is the reason why femtosecond lasers make use of a certain type of contact patient interface along with a suction ring, which holds the eye in a fixed position during the entire treatment. Among the several options, IntraLase femtosecond laser system makes use of a flat patient interface, which enables the system to be keratometry reading independent (Figs 3.3A and B).

Indeed, one of IntraLase femtosecond system main advantages is the efficiency in reducing the energy needed to create precise corneal incisions. Flat patient interface technology offers a unique depth positioning precision during planar incisions, which along with the laser technology, achieves an extremely precise positioning which optimizes treatment time and total energy delivered, being this a key factor when facing the wide variety of corneal transparency present in grafting surgery.

Due to this high precise positioning system, IntraLase created bubbles are not required to overlap each other as in other types of curved docking systems, but only to slightly create a communication channel as shown in Figures 3.4A and B. If positioning is not precise in a femtosecond laser, a tighter spot separation is usually performed to overcome the positioning tolerance, which will require the laser to place more spots than needed (high-degree of overlapping) to cover the treatment area, as well as increase the total energy due to the excess of laser firing. Selecting the proper spot separation will minimize both treatment time and total energy density per area, thus optimizing treatment time and early postoperative tissue response. Treatment time versus laser repetition rate can give an estimate on this femtolaser efficiency capability.

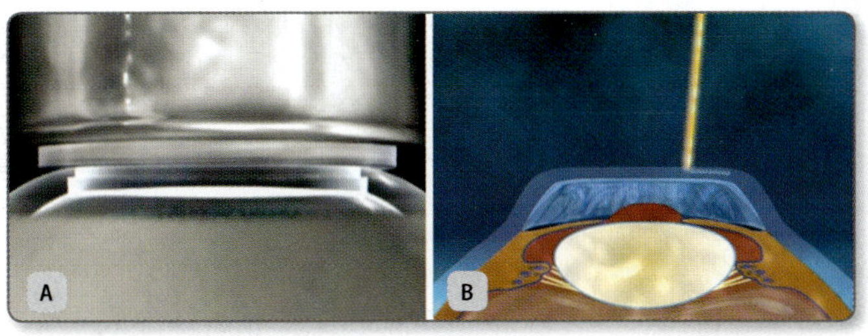

Figs 3.3A and B: K-Reading independency by the use of flat patient interface

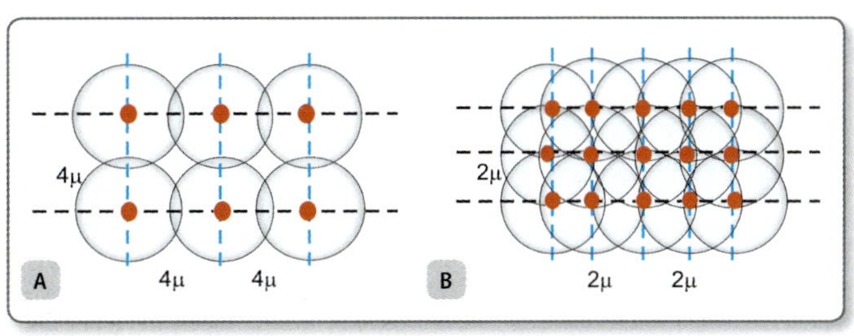

Figs 3.4A and B: (A) Efficient femtosecond energy and spot separation on IntraLase optimize both treatment time and total treatment energy density; (B) Whereas an excess on overlapping will increase total energy and enlarge treatment time and require higher repetition rates

Besides spot positioning and energy efficiency, the second main advantage of flat docking interface in IntraLase femtosecond laser consists in the ability to precisely adjust treatment positioning once suction and docking has been completed (Figs 3.5A and B), which enables the surgeon to overcome the challenging cases such us regrafting or arcuate keratotomy postkeratoplasty. Curved patient interfaces rely exclusively on mechanical centration during docking technique-losing part of the computer controlled precision typical from femtosecond lasers.

Mechanism to position every laser pulse is composed of three different positioning mechanisms X, Y and Z. Laser starts placing pulses from the deepest programed incision all the way up to the epithelial surface.

In conclusion, femtosecond laser technology precision offers the surgeon the ability to create identical diameter grafts between donor and recipient that can help to obtain higher visual acuity[2] and irregular astigmatism postoperative outcomes. Besides precision, this femtosecond laser is able to produce multiplanar self-healing profiles such as top-hat, mushroom or zigzag. This kind of graft edge profile provide better tissue coaptation, biomechanical stability helping to optimize clinical results, reduce the number of sutures and earlier suture removal[3-8] compared to mechanical procedure.

INTRALASE ENABLED KERATOPLASTY

IntraLase Enabled Keratoplasty Incision Design Software

IntraLase enabled keratoplasty (IEK) module is the designated incision design software related to corneal graft surgery in this specific femtosecond laser system. Corneal graft surgery comprises a huge variety of techniques, such as deep anterior lamellar keratoplasty (DALK), penetrating keratoplasty (PKP), Descemet's stripping automated keratoplasty (DSAEK) and others that require very different corneal graft profiles depending on the surgeon needs. Pattern design within IEK is based on a strictly open architecture strategy. As an architect would build a structure by using columns, beams and bricks, any corneal graft designed in IEK is comprised of simpler elements overlapping each other to form complex graft profiles as shown in Figures 3.5A and B.

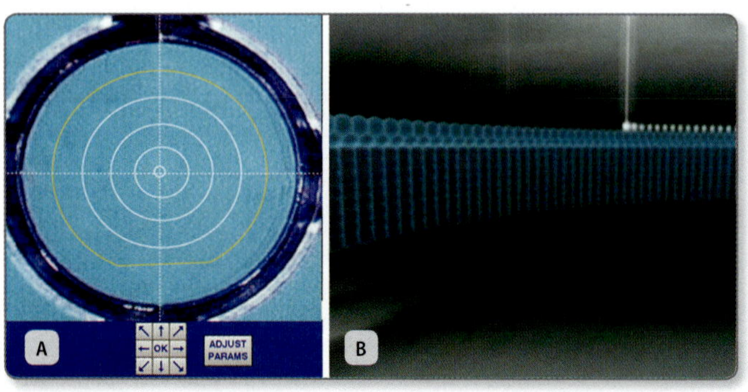

Figs 3.5A and B: (A) Software centration control system in IntraLase femtosecond laser. (B) Treatment where spots are placed starting from the deepest programed point to assure a clear pathway all the way up to epithelial surface

Within IEK incision design module, any corneal graft is designed as a combination of these single incisions as shown in Figure 3.6.

- Posterior side cut
- Anterior side cut
- Full lamellar cut
- Ring lamellar cut
- Alignment incisions.

Posterior Side Cut

Posterior side cut is a vertical cylindrical shaped incision with a certain diameter that starts from the base of the cornea at its posterior depth and extends up to meet the lamellar incision at the anterior depth point.

This posterior cylinder can be warped into a conic section by adjusting the side cut angle parameter as shown in the figure typically used in zigzag profiles (Fig. 3.7).

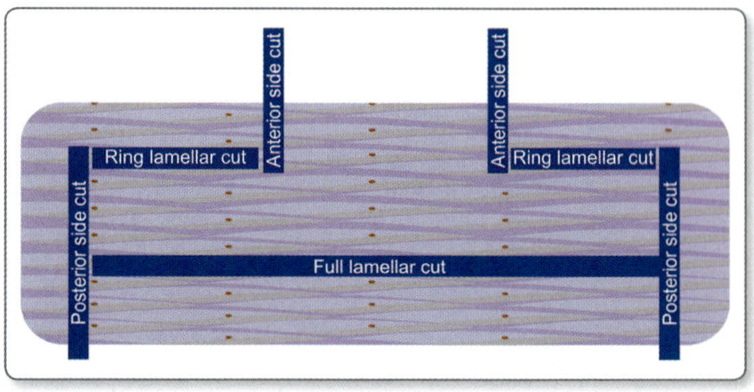

Fig. 3.6: Several simple incisions interact with each other to build a complex corneal graft

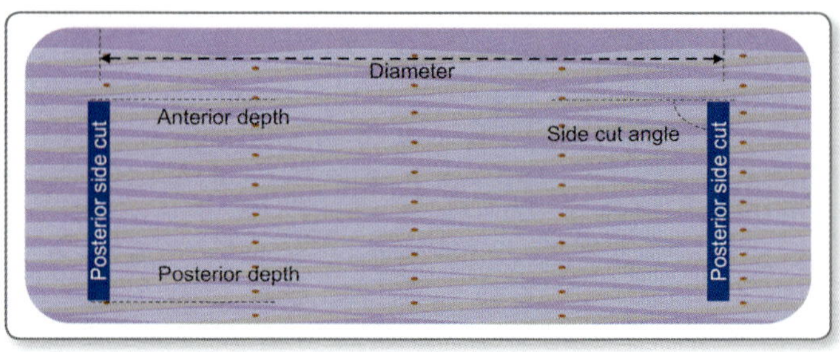

Fig. 3.7: Posterior side cut

Lamellar Cut

Lamellar cut is a planar incision parallel to the surface of the cornea that extends from the outer diameter to the inner diameter where is expected to meet the anterior side cut. This forms a ring incision whenever the inner diameter is present, and becomes a full lamellar incision with an inner diameter equals to zero (Fig. 3.8).

Anterior Side Cut

Anterior side cut is the analog section to posterior side cut, a cylindrical shaped incision that extends from the posterior depth to the surface of the cornea (Fig. 3.9). Anterior side cut is also used for astigmatic keratotomy to correct residual astigmatism following corneal graft surgery.

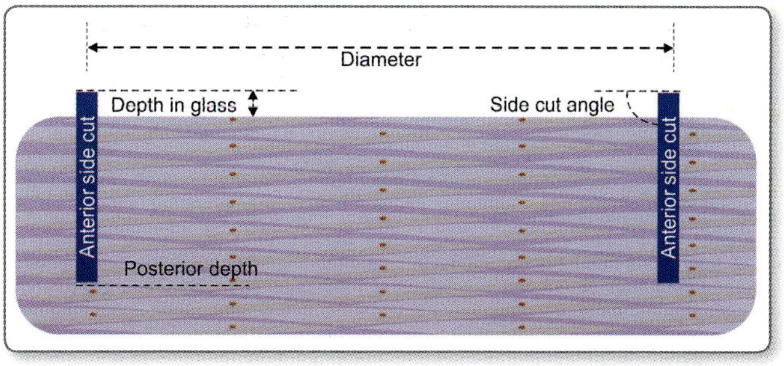

Fig. 3.9: Anterior side cut

Alignment Incisions

Alignment incision section is comprised of a series of radial incisions performed in both donor and recipient graft by the femtosecond laser. They are used by the surgeon as guide to match both grafts while suturing, and achieving a better torsional match, optimizing postoperative irregular astigmatism and visual acuity in lamellar grafts due to rotational alignment (Figs 3.10A and B).[2]

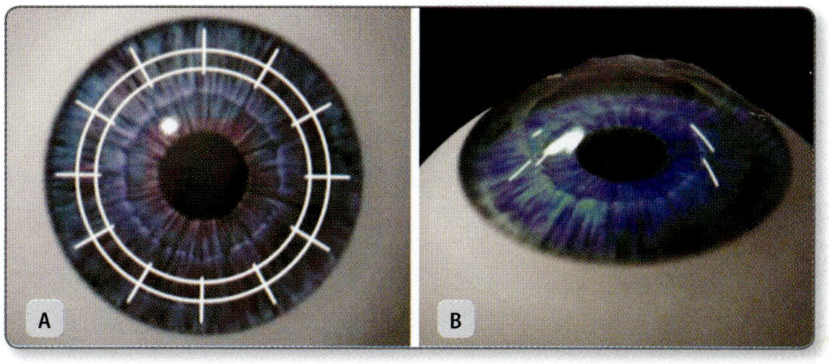

Figs 3.10A and B: (A) Radial incisions permit a correct graft alignment; (B) It helps in reducing irregular astigmatism

IntraLase Enabled Keratoplasty Incision Profiles

The combination of these previously introduced simpler incisions with IEK software produces a huge tool when designing the corneal graft, allowing the surgeon to produce tailored solutions to optimize clinical results on each different case. Posterior side cut, anterior side cut and lamellar cut can be combined in limitless number of complex edge profile graft combinations[10] with a very high level of precision in dimensions and centration which is not possible with other techniques.[9]

Several profiles have been extensively tested as shown in Figure 3.11, and it is up to surgeon needs to adapt them to the specific case scenario in the field of corneal graft surgery.

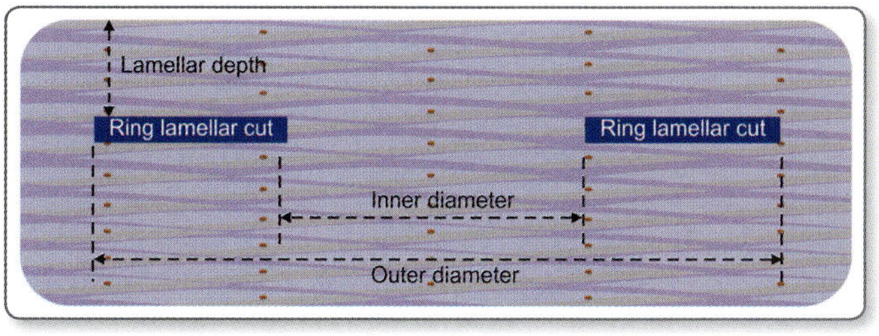

Fig. 3.8: Lamellar cut

It is needed however to understand from a deeper perspective the main characteristics of the basic profile architectures that can created in order to advance and obtain the full benefit of the design capabilities present in IEK module.

Top-Hat Based Edge Profile

The most instructional and well-known shape might be Top-hat profile, which is composed of three single steps imitating usual gentlemen hat morphology: (1) a wider posterior side cut; (2) ring lamellar cut; and (3) a narrower anterior side cut. This type of architecture maximizes the posterior tissue to the transplanted and may be better suited for posterior corneal disease, such as endothelial defect, Fuchs dystrophy or bullous keratopathy (Fig. 3.12).

Stepped incisions, such as top-hat were recognized long time ago to provide better wound healing response first by José Barraquer[12] and later by Busin.[13] Thus, self-healing profile grafts such as top-hat provide a superior tissue apposition, prevent wound leakage and can potentially accelerate wound healing.

Original top-hat incision uses 90º angulation as standard settings, and can evolve into different shapes by reducing the posterior side cut angle, such as square-zag

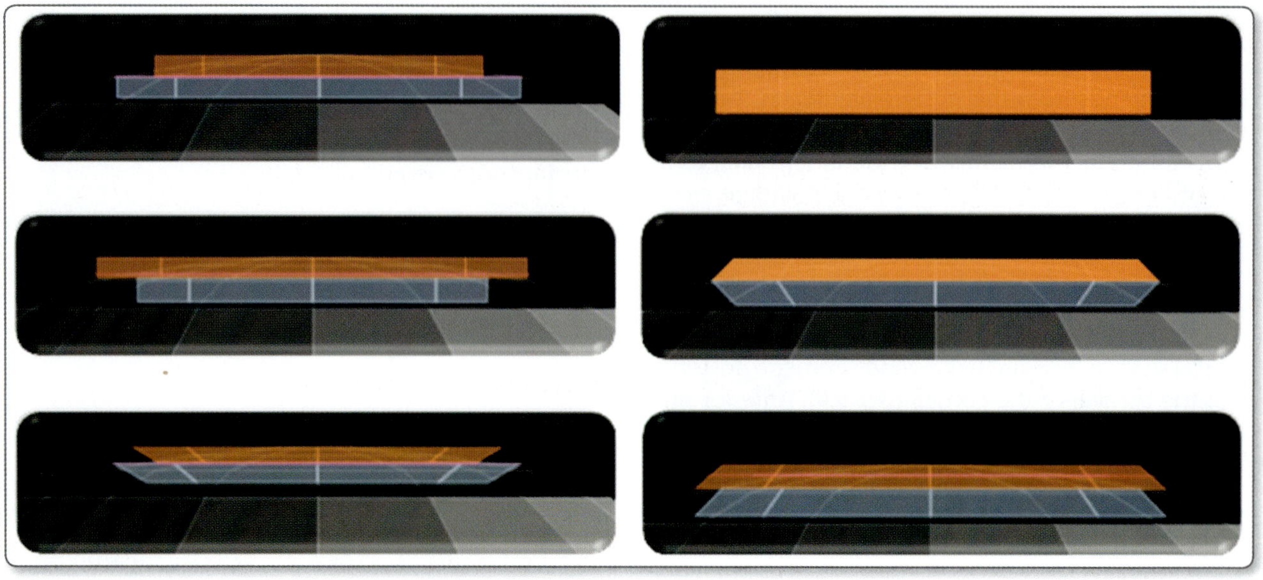

Fig. 3.11: Multiple IntraLase enabled keratoplasty (IEK) graft profiles

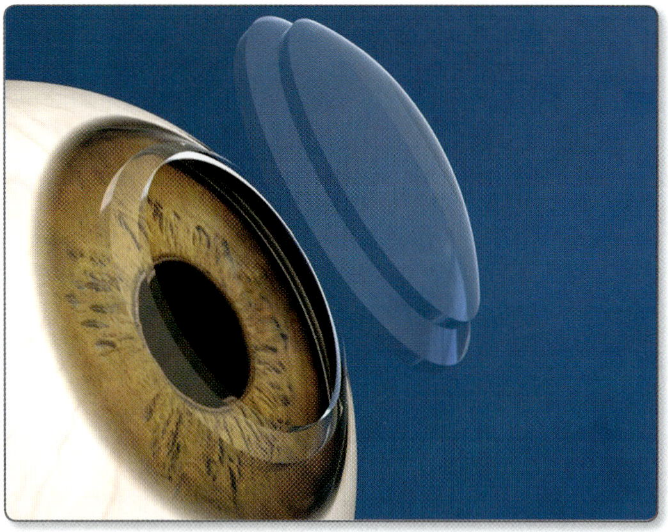

Fig. 3.12: Top-hat shaped graft

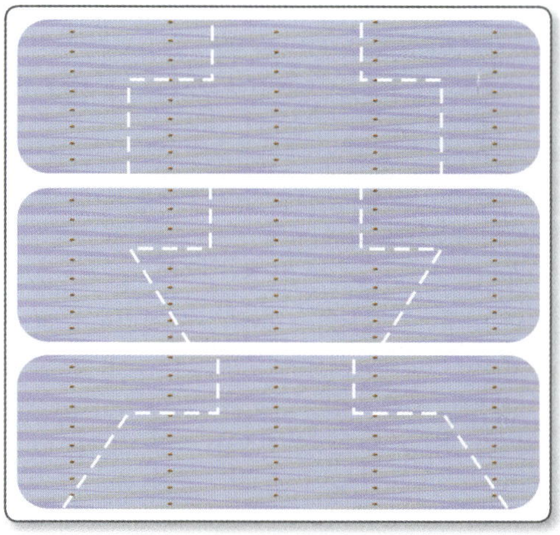

Fig. 3.13: Top-hat shaped graft (top), square-zag (middle), Flask (bottom)[10]

which reduces the deepest diameter which the objective of facilitating deep stromal dissection and direct visualization during deep lamellar surgery.[14]

By slating outwards the posterior side cut top-hat incision is known as Flask[9] and increases the posterior wound adhesion zone that can potentially improve wound healing (Fig 3.13).

Mushroom Based Edge Profile

The inverted version of a top-hat is known as mushroom and is often used for anterior surface surgery, being composed of a narrower posterior side cut and a wider anterior side cut both intersected by the ring lamellar cut. The broader anterior section maximizes superficial stromal area to the transplanted, which makes it more suitable to anterior lamellar corneal graft surgeries such as those caused by corneal burns or scarring, keratoconus or marginal pellucid degeneration. It is also an optimal approach to deep stromal anterior graft surgery because its morphology is optimized for direct visualization and access to posterior stroma during big bubble techniques.

Mushroom posterior side cut is typically angled at 90º and can be slanted outwards to improve the graft self-healing capabilities in several profiles as it is used in "Anvil" (Fig. 3.14).[11]

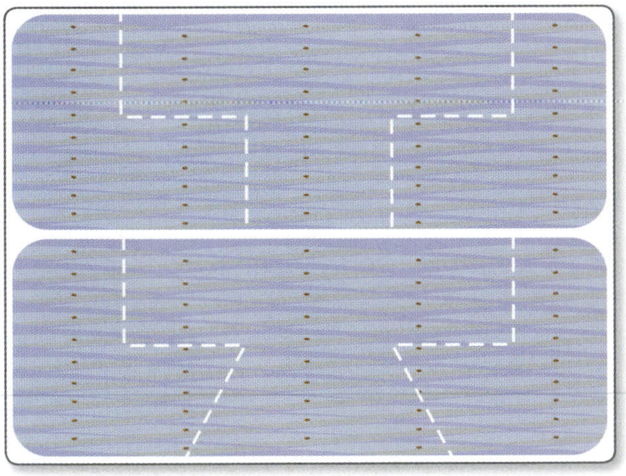

Fig. 3.14: Mushroom-shaped graft (top) and anvil configuration (bottom)[11]

Zigzag Based Edge Profile

One of the more complex edge profile incision is the zigzag graft, which compared to the squared angled profiles (top-hat, mushroom) presents superior biomechanical, sealing and coaptation properties.[10] On the downside, zigzag can be challenging in terms of configuration and graft handling due to its intrinsic configuration, which is the reason why it is considered a second step in the starting user learning curve.

Zigzag profile is composed of a slanted anterior and posterior side cuts connected by the ring lamellar cut. It can be adapted to maximize either anterior or posterior surface, which makes it suitable to a wide variety of situations. It is known as zigzag when the side cut angle is slanted inside the graft and Christmas tree when it is slanted outside the graft due to the morphological similarity to this seasonal tree (Fig. 3.15).

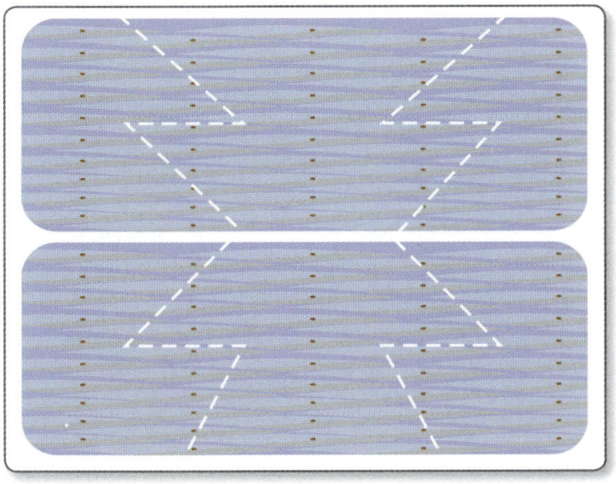

Fig. 3.15: Zigzag-shaped graft (top) and Christmas tree IEK profile (bottom)

Zigzag slanted incisions increase the wound apposition area, avoiding vertical cuts and offering superior biomechanical properties, as well as stronger wound healing and earlier postoperative period.[10] This angled incision profiles are also more forgiving in terms of depth matching, postoperatively.

Basics on Femtosecond Graft Architecture

Regardless of the profile, being used is of an important matter in terms corneal graft surgery designed with IntraLase, to understand the basics on femtosecond incisions and stepped graft architecture.

Incision Intersection

IntraLase-enabled keratoplasty corneal graft is formed by a combination of straight incisions, which need to interact which each other to obtain a clear and continuous graft profile that is easy to dissect, handle and be later extracted. Therefore, during profile design lamellar, posterior and anterior side cuts need to overlap with each other in both horizontal and vertical dimensions in order to assure laser incisions to communicate with each other.

Taking the well-known top-hat configuration as an example, anterior side cut is needed to end beneath the lamellar cut, whereas posterior side cut will start slightly superior to the lamellar shelf. This intersection assures the vertical continuity of the graft.

In the same way, lamellar cut outer diameter will be slightly superior to posterior side cut diameter whereas lamellar cut inner diameter has to be narrower than anterior side cut diameter providing the horizontal continuous incision.

The overlapping degree is generally set between 10 microns and 30 microns depending on the recipient cornea edematous state, opacities and treatment time needs. Highly edematous or opaque corneas can be harder to dissect especially if overlap is not set appropriately, whereas in clearer corneas overlap can be reduced to optimize treatment time (Fig. 3.16).

Lamellar Cut Depth

As stated previously, femtosecond graft profile can become a challenging procedure since every single case can be unique and tailored decisions may be needed on each individual case scenario. Moreover, corneal graft surgery is often the last resource to many corneal disorders such corneal ecstasia, supporting the need of a precise pachymetry map to approach the graft design and a complete understanding of graft architecture.

As a thumb rule, lamellar cut depth can be set to 50% of average pachymetry on a both donor and recipient normal

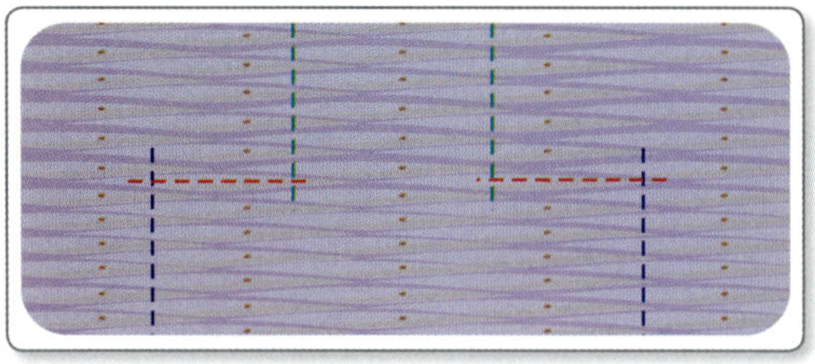

Fig. 3.16: Overlapping incisions

corneal hydration conditions. Lamellar cut will be then position half way from both anterior and posterior surfaces taking structural benefit from both cylinders at the same height.

Edematous recipient corneas must be taken carefully, as they will eventually come to normal depth after a successful corneal graft surgery once endothelial pump function is restored. In the same way, cultured corneas that may be expected to grow after corneal transplantation may be needed to be approached differently. Depending on the tissue depth evolution due to hydration changes, lamellar cut depth can be set slightly superior if shrinking may occur postoperatively, or on the other hand, it can be programed deeper if cultured corneas could expand after treatment.

Oversizing

Traditional corneal trephination has been extensively used, where donor grafts are typically obtained either with a punch block or with a trephined over the tissue coupled on artificial anterior chambers (AAC). On the recipient side, corneas in mechanical graft surgery are mostly cut with handled mounted trephines. On this type of surgery, incision angle compared to epithelial surface can be different depending on method being used,[10] and moreover, different keratometry readings will affect the graft edge-to-edge distance resulting in a donor versus recipient size and coaptation mismatch. It has also been of general use in corneal graft surgery to oversize the donor graft to achieve a better tissue apposition and refractive outcome due to the previously mention mechanical factors.

Femtosecond laser computer controlled precision is able to create identical sized grafts in terms of diameter regardless of the keratometry reading, which has led to recommend to use the exact same diameter in donor and recipient corneas,[10,11] improving tissue coaptation and postoperative visual results. It is then up to the surgeon to decide oversizing primarily just in terms of postoperative spherical refraction needs.

Deepest Posterior Point

Taking into account that oversizing is no longer needed in IntraLase corneal graft surgery, posterior depth on the posterior side cut might be the only parameter, which may present different settings in full thickness grafting.

When designing the donor graft in PKP, posterior depth must be set below maximum pachymetry reading in the incision area which enough depth to assure a clean and full thickness incision.

On the other hand, recipient might be moved from laser room to main surgical operating room. In these cases, patient movement makes it advisable to intentionally avoid performing a full thickness incision to prevent any pressure leaking during transportation from the Lasik room to the suturing surgical theater. Posterior depth is generally set 70 microns above the thinnest pachymetry reading point in the incision area, which is generally enough tissue to prevent wound leakage.[15]

This intentional safety gap composed of intact cornea, must be then opened by the surgeon by the use of a diamond knife, and then continue the graft circular profile with surgical scissors with caution to prevent any damage to the lamellar shelf.

SURGICAL PROTOCOL

Donor

IntraLase femtosecond corneal graft surgery requires the use of an AAC that holds donor tissue in proper position and pressure similar to a real patient during a Lasik procedure. Unlike mechanical keratoplasty in which trephines and punches are often used, AAC has certain restrictions regarding donor size, which makes it advisable ensure the eye bank will provide a donor cornea with enough scleral ring to fit and allow the AAC to be sealed properly without fluid leaks.

Besides the AAC, additional material needed during a femtosecond-assisted keratoplasty may include a sterile surgical field, forceps, three-way stopcock, balance saline solution (BSS), 10–20 cc syringe, intravenous (IV) bottle, viscoelastic, and an IntraLase patient interface (no suction ring is needed with the donor procedure).

Femtosecond corneal graft surgery is far from being a straightforward iterative procedure, but a complex design procedure, which makes every single procedure unique and different. Analyzing diagnostic data must be always within the surgical procedure protocol, such as recipient pachymetry and keratometry readings, white-to-white distance, patient anamnesis with special care to previous corneal graft surgeries and any corneal scars or opacities. Mechanical technique is usually full thickness or surgeon expertise dependent in terms of incision depth, however, with femtosecond lasers we are dealing with extremely precise incisional systems, which makes it necessary to dispose of a highly reliable pachymetry system if posterior cuts need to be done. Moreover, pachymetry readings can differ depending on the different systems available, especially on those recipient corneas undergoing a transplant surgery in advanced degenerative conditions making accurate pachymetry rather challenging, so it is highly recommended to cross-check in every case with intraoperative ultrasound pachymetry.

Once AAC is ready to use, donor tissue is transferred to from the sterile vial by gently grasping with forceps and then loaded on the chamber trying to avoid excess of BSS. Donor tissue centration must be checked carefully to optimize biomechanical graft matching and clinical outcomes, followed by an ink mark to assure laser precise centration and also handle any complication that may arise during the procedure (Fig. 3.17).

While transferring donor tissue to the AAC, bubbles beneath the donor tissue must be avoided to achieve a homogeneous tissue compression when docking the femtosecond laser patient interface, especially in non-penetrating procedures.

Artificial anterior chamber can be used either with an IV bottle or with a 10–20 cc syringe. If using a syringe it is advisable to engage a three-way stopcock to lock chamber when proceeding with the laser procedure, as laser docking can alter the syringe pressure depending on its size.

During the docking procedure, the previously placed ink mark should be followed in a precentering stage using X, Y and Z femtosecond system controls. Corneal contact will be indicated on upper right side of IntraLase laser screen as a green light and the usual docking meniscus. After contacting the corneal surface, X and Y controls must be avoided as they might induce irregular tissue compression and may lead to a non-circular graft. Once meniscus is clearly outside the programed graft area, Z movement might be stopped and no more mechanical movements are needed. Moreover is highly advisable for the surgeon to separate from both joystick and AAC or syringe to avoid any undesired movement.

At this point, in which no more hand movement is required, software centration must be used to precisely adjust X and Y position using the software centration arrows on the screen until treatment is perfectly aligned with previous corneal ink mark. Finally, from the laser procedure start users are encouraged not move during the treatment to avoid accidental movements on the AAC.

Artificial Anterior Chamber Pressure Management

Managing the pressure of AAC is one of the key elements on femtosecond corneal graft surgery learning curve. Either using an IV bottle or a syringe, the AAC pressure must be set between 55 and 65 mm Hg to assure a successful docking and a complete meniscus. In the end, target pressure should be similar to the level experienced clinically in a patient's eye under IntraLase femtosecond laser during the standard Lasik docking procedure.

Surgeon might make use of a portable tonometry system such as Barraquer tonometer to control the AAC pressure when donor tissue has been loaded the nearest possible to 55 mm of mercury (Fig. 3.18).

Setting a higher pressure than needed will produce a high tensional resistance that will prevent the full flattening of the cornea out of the treatment diameters, at the same time that a red light and continuous beep on the IntraLase device will advise of the maximum intraocular pressure is reached as seen in Figure 3.19. In case this event occurs, the user needs to undock the laser all the way up and readjust the AAC to a lower level.

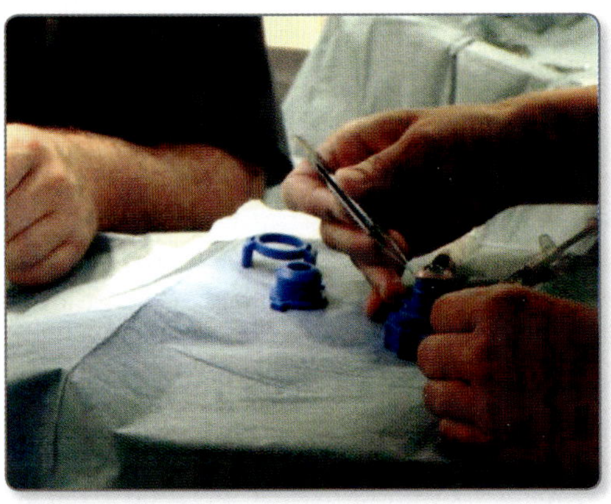

Fig. 3.17: Donor tissue is transferred to the artificial anterior chamber (AAC)
Courtesy: Blanca poyales

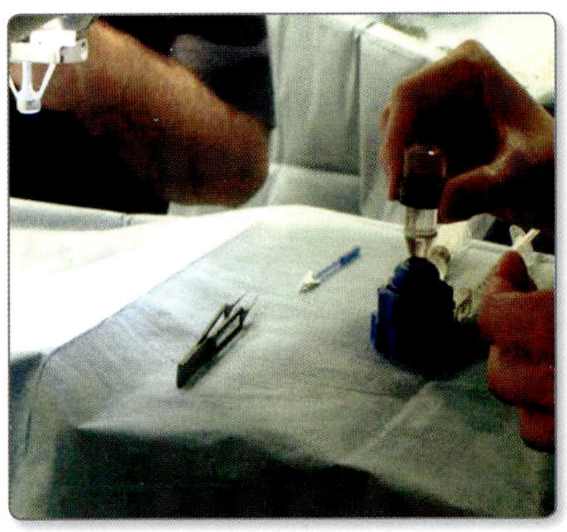

Fig. 3.18: Barraquer tonometer can be used to set AAC pressure to 55–60 mm Hg
Courtesy: Blanca poyales

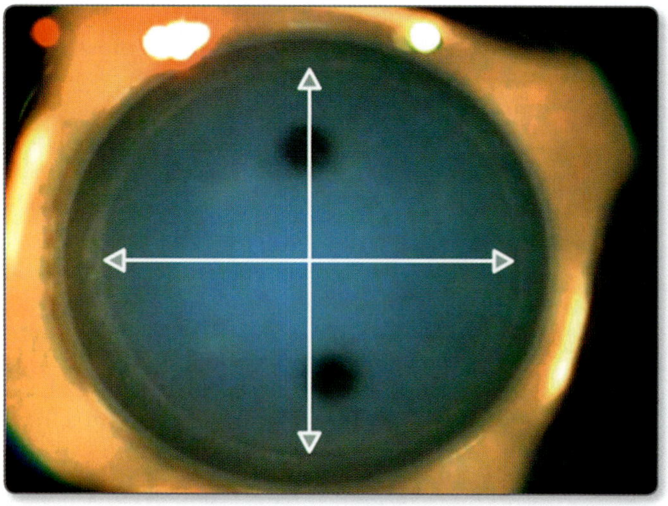

Fig. 3.19: Too high pressure on AAC can be detected when the meniscus is not expanding enough and IntraLase pressure control system activates the red light indicator

On the contrary setting a very low pressure might avoid the femtosecond laser to detect the corneal contact during the docking procedure, and thus, lock the safety mechanism that prevents the user to continue.

When using IV bottle, it is recommended to raise the bottle at least one meter above the height of the chamber during the docking procedure. After laser treatment, it is recommended to lower IV bottle height slightly over the AAC level to avoid an excess of saline salt solution pressure or "jet effect" in case of a full penetrating incision that could impact the laser internal objective and compromise the rest of the surgery.

If a syringe is being used, a three-way stopcock is mandatory to maintain pressure during the docking procedure in case if the AAC does not present its own sealing system. It will be comfortable to use a syringe size similar to 20 cc as the user will need a decent amount of BSS to mount the cornea and fill the AAC with. Once achieved the target pressure and before starting the docking procedure, the three-way stopcock must be closed sealing the chamber. After laser treatment, it is advisable to reopen the system and gently make a continuous infusion to prevent the chamber from collapsing.

Recipient

Femtosecond laser procedure and the rest of the corneal graft surgery involving graft extraction and suturing are generally done under different microscopes, even in different surgical rooms, which requires moving patient after the femtosecond laser treatment. This would be complicated in a full thickness graft is being performed, therefore it is necessary to leave a safety gap of posterior non-cut tissue on the recipient cornea which prevents any aqueous humor leakage during transportation.[15] At the same point, this safety gap reduces the complexity of femtosecond keratoplasty procedure on the recipient, which becomes relatively similar to a standard Lasik procedure.

Before starting the procedure, peribulbar or retrobulbar anesthesia should be administered with caution to avoid an uncontrolled increase in intraocular pressure or any conjunctival chemosis, which can prevent the suction ring to properly fixate the eye during the docking technique.

In the same way as the donor tissue, recipient surgical protocol starts by placing an ink mark on the targeted center of the graft. Docking and centration will be much more difficult on the recipient as the anesthesia will prevent the patient from collaborating, who can even present a decentered eyeball due the anesthesia. In order to overcome this situation, the ink mark and the software centration under the arrows screen become an enormous ally during the recipient procedure to achieve a proper centration.

Ink mark will be the reference to position the suction ring. Once the suction is applied, femtosecond laser should be lowered by twisting the joystick clockwise while holding the suction ring horizontal. After making the first corneal contact, X and Y movements should be avoided and only Z downward movement need to me made to complete the corneal flattening outside of the graft. It is an important matter to maintain the suction ring horizontal during the docking procedure to assure a homogeneous tissue contact with the patient interface, especially in advanced ecstasies or irregular topographies.

As soon as the meniscus is outside of the graft, suction ring must be locked and the surgeon might release both hands from the laser joystick and suction ring and make use of the software centration system to align with precision the graft to the ink mark position and start the laser treatment.

After treatment completion, suction is released and the patient is moved to the surgical microscope. It is important to remember cornea is still not fully penetrated.

Graft Manipulation

Recipient cornea transparency may have already been affected at the moment of corneal graft surgery. Therefore, femtosecond laser photodisruption can potentially leave corneal tissue adhesions at micron level, requiring that donor and recipient grafts are inspected cautiously to free any intralamellar bondings before extracting the graft. Graft will be always composed of several segments which the surgeon must follow 360º sequentially.

Using a top-hat configuration as an example, a Sinskey hook or similar instrument must be used by the surgeon to dissect the three incisions present in this stepped graft profile. First, it is needed to enter perpendicular to the surface of the cornea and find the anterior side cut, slide through the whole cylinder 360° and dissect anterior incision. Second, by twisting the Sinskey the doctor should find the lamellar cut, complete a 360° sweep, and proceed to the posterior side cut following the same strategy (Fig. 3.20).

The procedure is identical in both donor and receptor. However, recipient is not a full thickness cut which will be needed to finish first by opening with a diamond blade and continuing the circular incision with curved scissors with caution to avoid damaging the lamellar shelf.

Suturing

There is not a big difference between femtosecond corneal graft and mechanical surgery in terms of type of sutures being used so either single, running or double running sutures can be used at surgeon's discretion to minimize and control postoperative corneal astigmatism. Nonetheless, depth may play an important role in femtosecond graft suturing, as IntraLase stepped profiles must be sutured below the lamellar shelf to optimize wound healing and tissue coaptation.

In terms of healing response, any corneal graft whose posterior base is wider than the anterior base will produce a self-healing effect due to intraocular pressure outwards force that can lead to reduce the number of sutures and postoperative time, providing better wound stability[2-4,7] atttnd biomechanical results. In addition, slanted incision profiles such as zigzag can potentially offer superior sealing characteristics as they present a larger wound apposition area (Fig. 3.21).

AD-HOC CUSTOMIZATION

As in mechanical corneal graft surgery, femtosecond treatments need to be tailored to each specific case. IEK software will be programed differently in terms of number and type of incisions to be activated, dimensions,

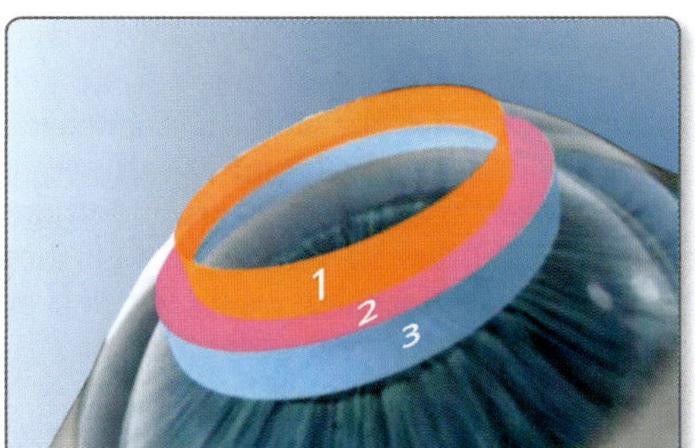

Fig. 3.20: Order to be followed when manipulating the femtosecond graft

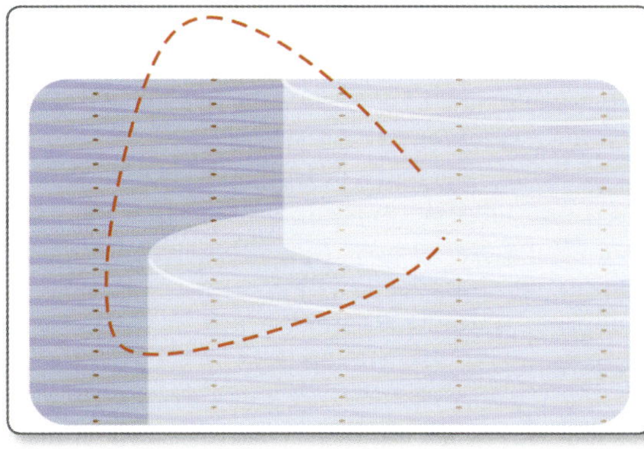

Fig. 3.21: Suturing the femtosecond corneal graft

energy and spot separation, what means the surgeon has great customization capabilities to overcome the most challenging cases.

Deep Stromal Anterior Keratoplasty

Being the most similar to Lasik technique, DALK femtosecond corneal graft surgery might be the starting point in the learning curve. When perforating surgery is not strictly needed, stromal anterior technique might be preferred by some surgeons because it can reduce tissue rejection by preserving corneal endothelium and better visual outcomes can be obtained presenting more regularity in terms of postoperative topography.[15]

Anterior side cut and lamellar incision are the two segments involved when designing anterior keratoplasty. Most common graft profile includes a side cut angle typically set with a 90° angulation due the simplicity of surgical graft handling (Fig. 3.22). As the surgeon advances in the learning curve, anterior side cut can be beveled-in, widening the graft base to increase wound apposition area and biomechanical stability, although this type of profile might be more difficult profile to dissect and handle.

When performing pre-Descemet techniques such as big bubble, special care must be taken regarding the side cut angulation as it can potentially prevent direct observation of the stromal surface on the periphery of the graft. Selecting a side cut angulation over 135° can become a challenge when

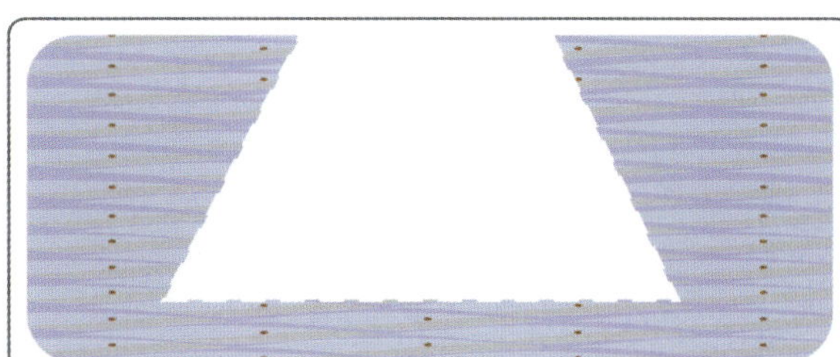

Fig. 3.22: Deep anterior stromal graft with beveled-in side cut angle

removing the edge portion of posterior stroma depending on the final graft depth.

Deep stromal graft surgery using big bubble technique offers great visual acuity postoperative outcomes, but presents a major drawback in terms of corneal perforation risk when needling during the Descemet search process. IntraLase femtosecond laser has been reported to help in overcoming this complication by adding a posterior channel, which communicates full lamellar cut in the direction of Descemet membrane as shown in Figure 3.23. This channel is done with the anterior side cut, using a tiny arcuate shaped incision, which extends from the lamellar cut down to 50 microns from corneal endothelium, therefore needing a highly reliable pachymetry system. Surgeon can latter use this channel, which has been tilted 30º from corneal plane to guide the cannula in a more precise way to place the bubble just above Descemet membrane, and can then reduce the learning curve and the risk of intraoperative corneal perforation.[15]

Penetrating Keratoplasty

Although penetrating corneal graft surgery has been extensively performed and is the most commonly used technique in corneal transplantation, it does still present very long postoperative period and in some cases, high postoperative astigmatism values.[16] Femtosecond Laser creates matching grafts with micron level precision that can potentially increase visual outcomes and visual rehabilitation.[5]

Within IEK module, penetrating graft surgery typically involves the use of a three stepped edge profile composed of anterior side cut, ring lamellar cut and posterior side cut. Depending on the bevel used in the side cut angle, different graft profiles can be obtained.

In terms of learning curve, top-hat or mushroom shapes can be easier to design and surgically handled, whereas slanted profiles such as zigzag can present higher challenges to the initial user.

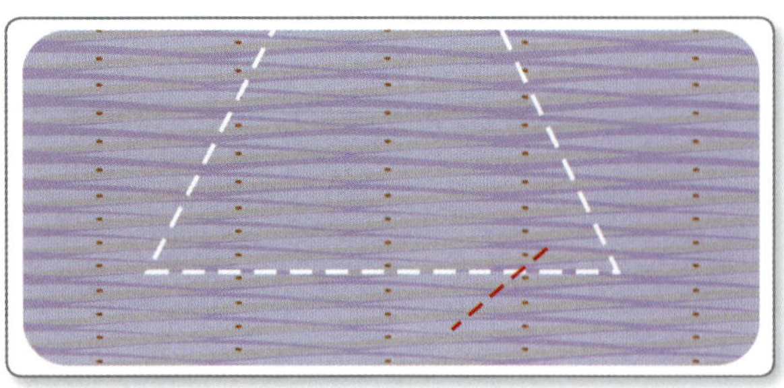

Fig. 3.23: Femto Descemet's stripping automated keratopalsty (DALK) graft and channel facilitating the access to Descemet membrane during big-bubble

Donor and recipient grafts are usually not oversized and the main difference resides on the deepest point, where donor is a full thickness graft whereas recipient is left with a safety gap, which minimizes the risk of pressure leak during patient transportation from Lasik room to the main operating room.

When complex profiles are used such as top-hat, mushroom or zigzag, lamellar cut depth is set to half of the average pachymetry reading from the graft diameter. Nonetheless, in case of highly edematous corneas, lamellar depth is usually programed at a shallower value to optimize depth matching on the anterior surface on the recipient due to the recovery of endothelial function and corneal rehydration process to normal state.

Penetrating keratoplasty is often left to the most advanced cases where corneal transparency might have been already severely affected. Strong opacities, keratopigmentation and similar conditions can attenuate Laser beam throughout and thus reducing the photodisruption effect resulting in an increase of stromal tissue microbridges complicating the graft dissection. In this situation, spot spacing shortening and energy increase can be adapted in IntraLase graft design screen to compensate for corneal opacities, up to 2 microns spot separation and a 90% of maximum energy.

When modifying spot separation, surgeon must acknowledge a treatment time increase and make sure it is not excessive in terms of intraocular pressure. Typical keratoplasty treatment times with 150 kHz iFS IntraLase device can vary from 25 to 45 seconds depending on corneal depth and spot spacing settings.

Deep Stromal Endothelial Keratoplasty

When only the endothelium has been damaged, posterior corneal graft surgery can be considered as an alternative to PKP. Posterior techniques leave the surface of the recipient cornea not affected, thus reducing the risk of infections and postoperative astigmatism. The use of femtosecond Laser reduces the risk of endothelial loss due to tissue manipulation and trephination and can potentially obtain more predictable graft thickness, which can reduce complications related to shallow anterior chamber depths.[17]

Both posterior side cut and full lamellar cut are activated within IntraLase design software during posterior lamellar corneal graft surgery. It is of special interest the spot separation and energy setting as they can play an important factor in stromal bed quality, which is optimized by selecting the lowest energy and spot spacing that allows graft dissection.

Graft thickness is also a key factor in the success of endothelial graft surgery.[18] A thicker graft will be easier to handle and avoid graft folding, while a thinner graft can potentially offer fewer complications in shallow anterior chamber depths, less hypermetropic shift and better structural properties. Donor graft thickness is set in the lamellar cut depth parameter, by subtracting the desired central graft depth from donor central corneal pachymetry reading.[19]

Both recipient and donor can be created with femtosecond laser, which increases wound healing and reduces the chance of graft dislocation.[17] However, manual descemetorhexis using a reverse Sinskey hook can also be used in the recipient cornea, although the graft diameter matching can be compromised.

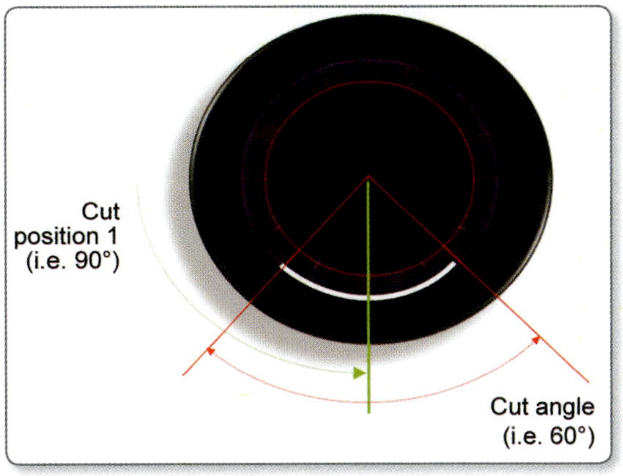

Fig. 3.24: Superior arcuate incision (cut position 1 = 90º) with a length corresponding to 60º (white)

Astigmatic Keratotomy Postcorneal Graft Surgery

High astigmatism is usually present in postoperated patients who have undergone penetrating graft surgery mainly due to graft diameter and depth mismatch, and irregular forces coming from the suturing procedure.[19,20] It can generate severe visual disturbances and can be reduced by postoperative arcuate incisions.

Mechanical technique is carried out with a diamond blade with poor predictability and stability in terms of refraction and several complications such as corneal perforation[21] possibly influenced by the lack of incision reproducibility, uniformity and precision.[20] Femtosecond laser offers a precise positioning, depth, uniformity and reproducibility of incisions that might potentially increase technique reproducibility and results,[19-21] as well as a potential reduction in epithelial ingrowth by the lack of mechanical blade penetration.

IntraLase-enabled arcuate keratotomy capabilities are included in the anterior side cut standard parameters. The user can control positioning, depth, diameter of the incision, as well as independent axis and width settings for separate arcuate incisions under the parameters known as cut position and cut length (measured in degrees or arc) as shown in Figure 3.24.

Similar to intracorneal ring segments and other astigmatic correction treatments, arcuate incisions predictability are affected by treatment centering.[22] It is then required of a precise centration within the visual axis to assure good postoperative outcomes. The user is encouraged not to leave centration to the likely willing patient fixation ability, but to place a careful ink mark in the desired optical zone target and precisely align the treatment with the laser centration software once docking has been completed.

A precise and reliable pachymetry system is required to perform femtosecond arcuate incisions, and a depth of 80% is generally set as standard procedure, which might produce a slight inferior correction effect compared to the full depth mechanical nomograms.

IntraLase femtosecond laser procedure is always started from the posterior side all the way up to the surface, giving the surgeon the opportunity to inspect for any depth calculation disparity. The use of arcuate femtosecond laser allows the surgeon to abort the treatment in case of an overestimation of corneal depth before the incision is completed. In case depth has been overestimated, it can be easily detected by the user by the lack of any corneal incision during the first treatment seconds. Instead, micro-bubbles corresponding to spots in the aqueous humor appear dispersed trough the expected incision location. This gives the user the ability to abort the treatment before a full thickness penetration, and recheck pachymetry and depth settings.

DISCLOSURE

Juan Gabriel Ortiz is the clinical development manager for IMEX, current distributor of Abbot Medical Optics in Spain and Portugal.

REFERENCES

1. Faktorovich EG. Femtodynamics: A guide to laser settings and procedure techniques to optimize outcomes with femtosecond lasers. Slack Incorporated; 2009.
2. Villarrubia A, Mendicute J, Pérez Santonja JJ, et al. Queratoplastia Lamelar. Técnicas Quirúrgicas. Comunicación Solicitada 81 Congreso de la Sociedad Española de Oftalmología. Mac Line SL; Madrid: 2005.
3. Birnbaum F, Wiggerman A, Maier PC, et al. Clinical results of 123 femtosecond laser-assisted penetrating keratoplasties. Graefes Arch Clin Exp Ophthalmol. 2013;251:95-103.

4. Birnbaum F, Maier P, Reinhard T. Perspectives of femtosecond laser-assisted keratoplasty. Ophthalmologe. 2011,108:807-16.
5. Ignacio TS, Nguyen TB, Chuck RS, et al. Top hat wound configuration for penetrating keratoplasty using the femtosecond laser: a laboratory model. Cornea. 2006;25:336-40.
6. Maier P, Böhringer D, Birnbaum F, et al. Improved wound stability of top-hat profiled femtosecond laser-assisted penetrating keratoplasty in vitro. Cornea. 2012;31:963-6.
7. Cheng YY, Tahzib NG, van Rij G, et al. Femtosecond laser-assisted inverted mushroom keratoplasty. Cornea. 2008;27:679-85.
8. Chan CC, Ritenour RJ, Kumar NL, et al. Femtosecond laser-assisted mushroom configuration deep anterior lamellar keratoplasty. Cornea. 2010;29:290-5.
9. Sarayba MA, Maguen E, Salz J, et al. Femtosecond laser keratome creation of partial thickness donor corneal buttons for lamellar keratoplasty. J Refract Surg. 2007;23:58-65.
10. Farid M, Kim M, Steinert RF. Results of penetrating keratoplasty performed with a femtosecond laser zigzag incision initial report. Ophthalmology. 2007;114:2208-12.
11. Price FW, Price MO. Femtosecond laser shaped penetrating keratoplasty: One-year results utilizing a top-hat configuration. Am J Ophthalmol. 2008;145:210-4.
12. Barraquer JI. Technique of penetrating keratoplasty. Am J Ophtalmol. 1950;33:6-17.
13. Busin M. A new lamellar wound configuration for penetrating keratoplasty surgery. Arch Ophthalmol. 2003;121:260-5.
14. Neuhann TF, Lege BB, Joergensen JS, et al. Femtosecond laser profiled penetrating Keratoplasty with the IntraLase FS60 IEK. Chicago: ASCRS; 2008.
15. McAllum P, Kaiserman I, Bahar I, et al. Femtosecond laser top hat penetrating keratoplasty: wound burst pressures of incomplete cuts. Ach Ophthalmol. 2008;126:822-5.
16. Buzzonetti L, Petrocelli G, Valente P. Femtosecond laser and big-bubble deep anterior lamellar keratoplasty: a new chance. J Ophthalmol. 2012;264590.
17. Kook D, Derhartunian V, Bug R, et al. Top-hat shaped corneal trephination for penetrating keratoplasty using the femtosecond laser: a histomorphological study. Cornea. 2009;28:795-800.
18. Monterosso C, Fasolo A, Caretti L, et al. Sixty-kilohertz femtosecond laser-asisted endothelial keratoplasty: clinical results and stromal bed quality evaluation. Cornea. 2011;30(2):189-93.
19. Prakash G, Agarwal A, Jacob S, et al. Femtosecond-assisted descemet stripping automated endothelial keratoplasty with fibrin glue-assisted sutureless posterior chamber lens implantation. Cornea. 2010;29:1315-9.
20. Buzzonetti L, Petrocelli G, Laborante A, et al. Arcuate keratotomy for high postoperative keratoplasty astigmatism performed with the IntraLase femtosecond laser. J Refract Surg. 2009;25:709-14.
21. Kymionis GD, Yoo SH, Ide T, et al. Femtosecond-assisted astigmatic keratotomy for post-keratoplasy irregular astigmatism. J Cataract Refract Surg. 2009;35:11-3.
22. Bahar I, Levinger E, Kaiserman I, et al. IntraLase-Enabled Astigmatic Keratotomy for postkeratoplasty astigmatism. Am J Opthalmol. 2008;146:897-904.

Chapter

4

Therapeutic Procedures Using the VICTUS™ Femtosecond Laser Platform

Tobias Neuhann

CHAPTER OUTLINE

- Key technical features of the VICTUS femtosecond laser platform
- Description of the development and evolution of the VICTUS technology
- Diagnostic imaging technology
- Benefits of curved corneal interface in the VICTUS system
- Intelligent pressure sensor as a control of eye fixation
- Control of eye stability and monitoring process during the procedure
- Technical profile of the 160 kHz platform

Corneal grafting surgery technique:

- Penetrating keratoplasty (40 to 80 kHz)
- Patterns profile´s selection
- Decagon cut designs gives 33% more contact surface
- Surgical application details
- Outcomes
- Deep anterior lamellar grafts
- Endothelial keratoplasty/Posterior lamellar grafts
- Additional procedures performed with Technolas femtosecond laser
- Analysis of cost effectiveness

INTRODUCTION

More than 100 years[1] of experience with corneal lamellar and perforating keratoplasty have shown a frequent increase in astigmatism even after suture removal. For this reason, calls for a corneal trephine and incision system to ensure tensionless symmetrical corneal surgery have arisen for a long time. Watertight congruent cut edges as well as trephination from epithelial to endothelial are additional requests.[2]

The introduction of the femtosecond laser and especially the Technolas Femtec laser has been an almost perfect answer to these basic requirements, however, not in a way as formulated back then. We thus experience a paradigm change, as often found in the past years in ophthalmology. The platform developed and manufactured by Bausch + Lomb/Technolas Perfect Vision (Rochester, NY and Munich, Germany) is unique among femtosecond lasers available today due to its versatility.

While the company's initial focus was on therapeutic indications, including intrastromal corneal ring segment (ICRS) tunnels for keratoconus and penetrating keratoplasty, this femtosecond laser system has evolved over time to include a wide range of applications (Table 4.1). These include an intrastromal presbyopia treatment (INTRACOR) in 2009, followed by the incorporation of femto-cataract procedures in 2011, when the companies launched the VICTUS® femtosecond laser platform in November 2011. The VICTUS received US 510 (k) Food and Drug Administration (FDA) clearance for LASIK flaps and anterior capsulotomy in August 2012. With the ability to perform cataract surgery and therapeutic corneal procedures, as well as creation of flaps for laser in-situ keratomileusis, the VICTUS femtosecond laser platform is an excellent tool for the anterior segment surgeon (Fig. 4.1). Author's personal experience using a femtosecond laser for therapeutic indications, such as corneal grafts is based upon using the Technolas 520 F model, the previous generation of this laser system.

Table 4.1: Evolution of the B+L/VICTUS femtosecond laser system

Year	*Event*
2004	FDA 510(k) clearance and CE mark for LASIK flap
2005	First ICRS tunnels for keratoconus
2005	First astigmatic keratotomy cuts
2005	First penetrating keratoplasty
2006	First posterior lamellar keratoplasty
2007	First noncircular decgon-shaped KP
2007	First link between femtosecond laser and diagnostic unit
2007	First intrastromal refractive procedures (INTRACOR)
2009	INTRACOR recives CE Mark
2011	VICTUS receives CE Mark
2012	VICTUS receives 510(k) FDA clearance for LASIK flaps and anterior capsulotomy

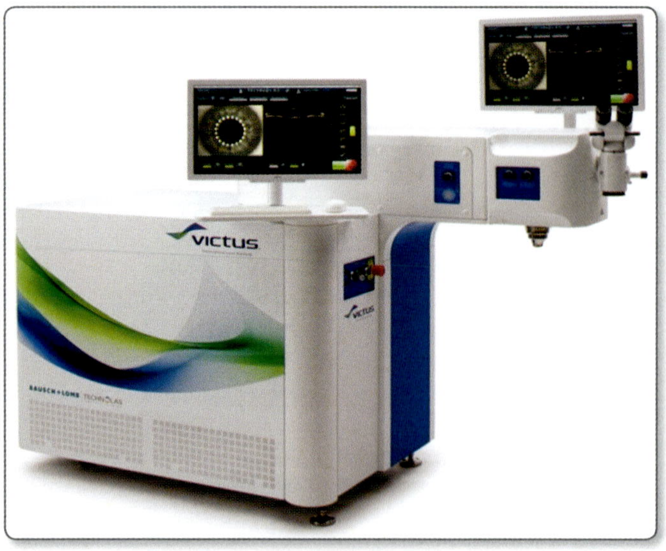

Fig. 4.1: VICTUS™ femtosecond laser platform

KEY FEATURES OF THE VICTUS FEMTOSECOND LASER PLATFORM

The design elements that enable the VICTUS™ femtosecond laser platform to perform different procedures, including the therapeutic indications are:

- A unique optical system
- Curved patient interface: This is designed to reduce applanation of the cornea and minimize corneal folds to allow a straight laser path during the cutting of corneal tissue. TPV was the first company to develop a curved patient interface for corneal surgery with a femtosecond laser. The curved patient interface is designed to provide gentle eye fixation with minimal corneal deformation (Figs 4.2 and 4.3).
- Intelligent pressure sensors: These sensors ensure optimal pressure for all procedures by using three-dimensional (3D) eye force/pressure evaluation. The multiple, highly sensitive sensors enable pressure monitoring and control in 3D (Fig. 4.4). This minimizes distortion and avoids corneal folds or ripples, which is particularly advantageous when performing corneal grafts. The sensors also enable the surgeon to center and stabilize the eye with the appropriate pressure for the procedure.

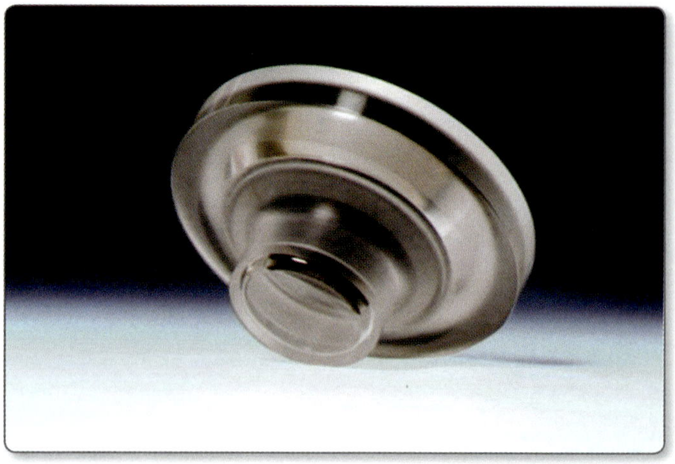

Fig. 4.2: TPV curved patient interface

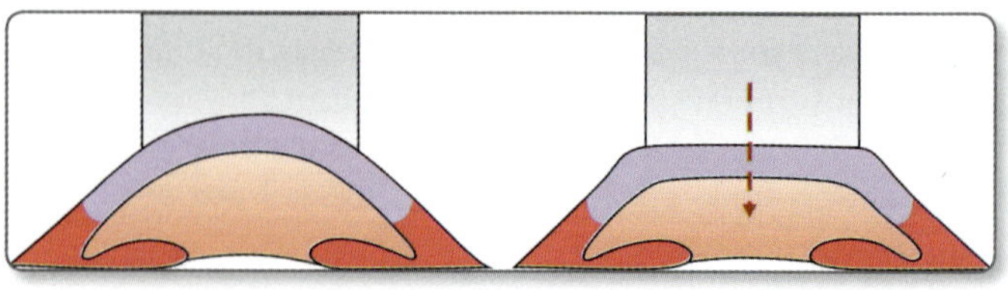

Fig. 4.3: The TPV femtosecond laser patient interface in comparison to IntraLase patient interface

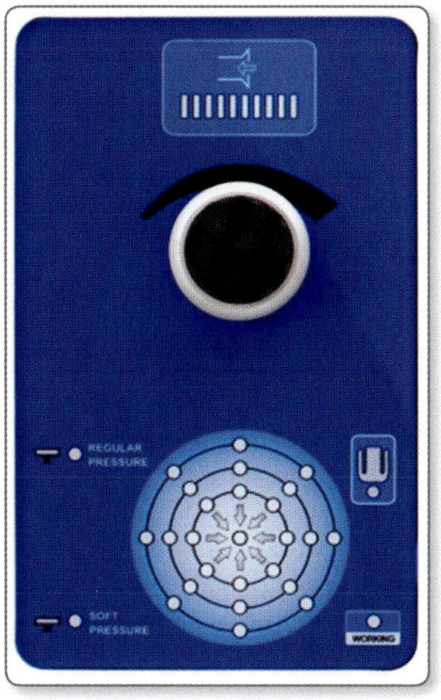

Fig. 4.4: Intelligent pressure control

- Eye stability and monitoring: The adjustable vacuum maintains necessary suction when the eye is docked, which optimizes eye stability for all procedures.
  - The combination of curved patient interface, pressure sensors, along with the eye stability and monitoring enable the Technolas femtosecond laser to precisely engage the curved interface to the patient's eye, depending on the type of the procedure.
- Faster pulse rate: The system is capable of multiple pulse settings ranging up to 160 kHz (Table 4.2).
- Graphic user interface (GUI): The new system also features a user-friendly graphical software interface for easy treatment planning and monitoring based on the ocular data obtained through continuous optical coherence tomography (OCT) imaging (Fig. 4.5).

INTERFACE

The difference between the Technolas Femtec workstation, and that of the IntraLase femtosecond laser, in addition to various technical details, is mainly the contact pressure exerted on the patient´s interface (Figs 4.2 and 4.3). While

Table 4.2: Pulse rate settings based on indication for the VICTUS platform	
Treatment	*VICTUS pulse rates*
Cataract	80 kHz
Lasik flap	160 kHz
Intracor	40 kHz
Therapeutic	80 kHz

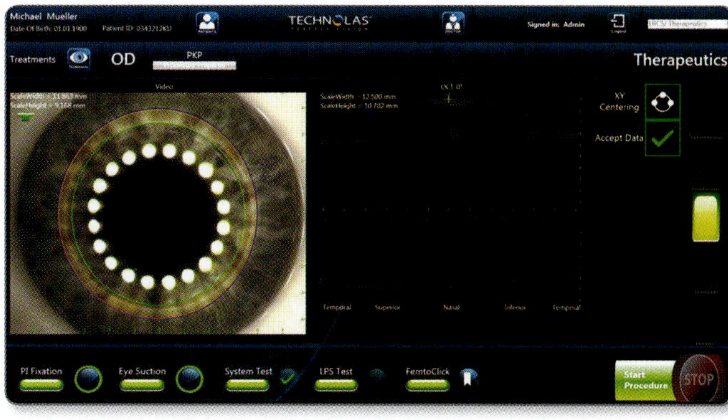

Fig. 4.5: Graphic user interface with real-time, high contrast OCT
Abbreviation: OCT—optical coherence tomography

the IntraLase femto laser requires full flattening of the cornea and of the interface, the cornea is not flattened when using the Technolas femto laser, since the interface is curved. The spherical interface is especially valuable in patients with severe keratoconus. The decisive advantage is firstly the considerably lower intraocular pressure increase and secondly cut along the naturally curved cornea. Also femtosecond lasers belonging to the new generation use this principle of the spherical interface in the treatment of cataract because of the lower induced pressure increase. The importance of this criterion is an aspect to be investigated in larger studies in the future.

THERAPEUTIC PROCEDURES

The author's experience with the therapeutic software modules on the Technolas femtosecond laser is:

- Descemet's endothelial keratoplasty
- Intrastromal ring segments (intracorneal ring segments; ICRS) implantation
- Arcuate cuts for astigmatic keratotomy (AK)
- Penetrating and lamellar keratoplasty (PKP and DALK)
- Corneal crosslinking.

In this chapter, the author will cover three of these procedures: PKP, as well as anterior and posterior lamellar grafts. In addition, in the accompanying box, we include some information regarding the other therapeutic procedures performed with the laser.

PENETRATING KERATOPLASTY

Although the first mechanical trephine systems trephined the donor transplant from endothelial to epithelial and the recipient from epithelial to endothelial, newer trephine systems, such as the guided trephine system (GTS) of Krumeich or Moria are able to cut the donor as well as the recipient tissue from the outside to the inside under almost identical conditions using an artificial anterior chamber. Author uses the same artificial anterior chamber system of the GTS to obtain the donor transplant with the Femtec workstation. The laser cuts from endothelial to epithelial, i.e. from the inside to the outside! At present, this is only possible with the help of a femtosecond laser! For this purpose, the Femtec laser employs a spherical interface applying low pressure and a selectable cutting speed between 40 kHz and 80 kHz, a pulse duration of 600 fs and a pulse energy of less than equal to 4 µJ. At average, the entire preparation takes about 90 seconds. Vital criteria for the cut quality are the selection of the horizontal and vertical spacing as well as the preset energy that needs to be determined for the individual device.

For PKP, the Technolas femtosecond laser software is fully customizable in terms of bed styles, rim shape (circular, top-hat, mushroom) and rim style (circular, orientation teeth and decagon). The software also allows peripheral marking, plus precise depth and diameter selection including a software predictor for anterior and posterior diameter and adjustable step depth for top-hat and mushroom shapes.

When first starting with corneal graft procedures using a femtosecond laser, it is helpful to familiarize yourself with the laser by practicing with pig eyes. Optimal centration and docking of the curve patient interface is essential, but the learning curve is relatively short owing to the use of the intelligent pressure sensors. Correct docking is also essential to minimize the presence of corneal folds, as well as careful planning of the procedure based upon topographic data.

When performing PKP, it is important to obtain reliable and comparable pachymetry data on both the transplant and the recipient cornea. In most cases, the initial incision depth starts with a setting of 1,300 µm. During the planning process, the outcome of the desired posterior cut and not the anterior diameter will be calculated and then a slightly larger donor cut (200 µm) will be created to reduce both surgically induced astigmatism and Descemet folds.

The author achieved the best results with the so-called double pass application: The first cutting cycle ends 150 µm below the epithelial surface of the transplant as well as of the recipient, and the second cycle using the same settings ends 150 µ above the epithelium, i.e. in the PMMA interface. In this way, the individually desired residual strength of the cut corneal slice to be eventually prepared and removed in the operating room is obtained without having to change the settings of spacing and energy.

CUT DESIGN

The known cut designs, such as top hat, mushroom, zigzag, Christmas tree, zig square, barrel, etc. have one thing in common—they all are round. Owing to its innovative scanner the Femtec laser also allows angular cut edges in addition to these known designs. Currently, author is working with a decagonal cut design (Figs 4.6A and B). Additionally, the cut edges are not vertical but rather at 60°, which corresponds to a 33% surface enlargement of the cut edges.

VARIABLE DIAMETER

Another advantage of the femtosecond laser in corneal transplantation is the nearly unlimited variety of donor and recipient transplant diameters. Theoretically, this was also possible with the mechanical trephines; however, the precision of 0.1 or 0.2 mm never was as perfect as that offered by the Femtec laser. Author currently uses a 0.2 mm oversizing of the transplant even with decagon cuts, which almost perfectly meets the old demand for wound tightness. Whether the next steps will be stronger or customized, oversizing will become clear once surgeons are able to interoperatively measure sphere, cylinder, bulb length and wave fronts. Corresponding developments are currently being intensely worked on by others.

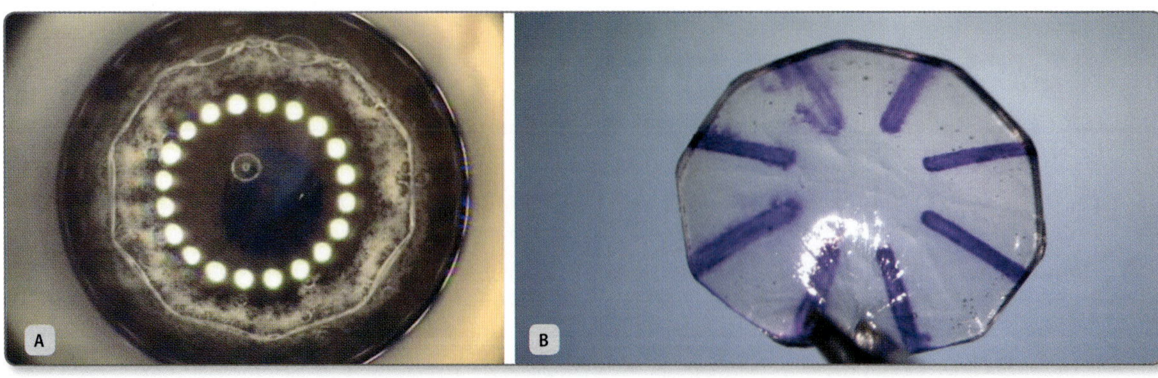

Figs 4.6A and B: Decagonal keratoplasty procedure and transplant

SHAPE DESIGN

In 1963, Barraquer[3] published an angular cut design in keratoplasty. The problem back then was especially the reproducibility of the manually prepared congruency of the cut edges. Barraquer was very early to recognize the advantage of the angular transplant, i.e. the edges mostly prevent transplant distortion. Forty years later, Busin also described the advantages of an edge design for corneal transplantation.[4] With round transplants, distortion frequently occurs due to the continuous suturing technique, so that the time-consuming single-stich technique is still favored. With angular grafts, the continuous suture can be used with the perfectly congruent corners ideally preventing torque (Fig. 4.7). This, in turn, is reflected by improvement of the clinical results.

The author has been using the decagon shape since 2008 and report here on his 2-year results of 21 eyes that underwent PKP using a decagonal approach with the Technolas femtosecond laser.

CAUSE FOR KERATOPLASTY

Of the patients included in this follow-up, 11 had advanced keratoconus without an intact Descemet membrane. In the remaining 10 eyes, seven had pseudophakic bullous keratopathy, two had undergone unsuccessful Descemet's stripping endothelial keratoplasty (DSEK) transplantation procedures and one had a decompensated cornea following a crosslinking procedure.

SURGICAL TECHNIQUE

To prepare the donor cornea, author had performed a decagonal trephination that was 0.2 mm larger than the opening created in the recipient cornea—for example, if the diameter of the cornea graft was 8.1 mm, than the receiver bed opening was programed for 7.9 mm. The cutting edges were inclined 60° to the inside. For the artificial anterior chamber, author used a modified version of the GTS Krumeich trepan systems. For the receiver bed, he created a decagonal cut that also had a 60° angulation.

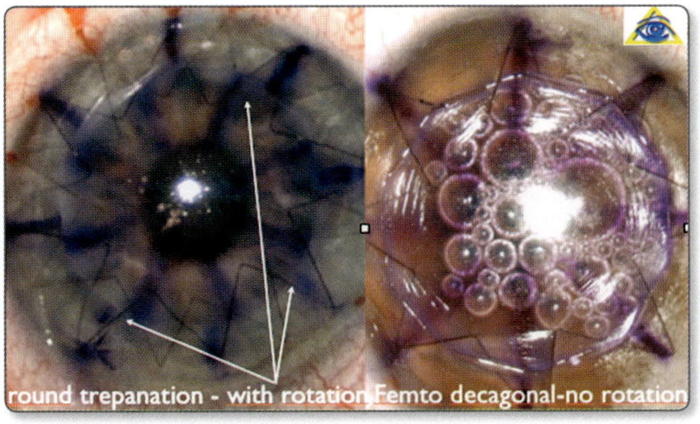

Fig. 4.7: The marks on the donor transplant have rotated inadvertently while the marks on the decagon transplant stayed perfectly in place

The suture technique that was used, which remains the greatest variable when performing a corneal transplant, was essentially the same as what author had used for manual keratoplasty procedures: two running sutures with eight external fixation points. The first suture was a continuous suture using 10/0-ethilon, while for the second suture; 11/0-nylon was used. This approach can be used because of the approximately 33% greater stromal surface for wound healing that is available due to the 60° angulation of the cut. The 10 corners of the graft result in a uniform distribution of the donor cornea to the recipient bed. Clinical observation has shown that 11/0-nylon induces less astigmatism than 10/0 in 80% of cases. The author tends to remove the 10/0 suture no later than 6-month postoperative and leave the 11/0 suture in place. His clinical impression after 36-month of experience with the decagon technique is that the corneal healing process seems to be much faster and watertight than with the manual technique.

In addition to the reduced level of astigmatism, the 60° cutting angle makes the suturing process more straightforward because the corresponding depth of cut between donor and recipient is significantly easier to locate under the microscope. Another advantage of the decagonal approach is that the corners appear to help stabilize the graft (Fig. 4.7).

VISUAL RESULTS

The corrected visual acuity at 6 months postoperative averaged 0.36 ± 0.6 D (Fig. 4.8). But more noteworthy were the astigmatism results—both the corneal topography and manifest refraction showed a mean astigmatism 1.8 ± 1.2 D (range of 0.5 and 4.25 D). All eyes had a relatively fast visual recovery result. This is by far better than our results with the manual technique and statistically relevant (Figs 4.9 and 4.10).

At 12 months postoperative, there was an average endothelial cell loss of 12.5%. However, because the donor endothelial cell count provided by different eye banks is higher than what was measured, we do not think this rate of cell loss is of concern.

COMPARISON OF THE RESULTS WITH PUBLISHED DATA

If we compare our results with previously published studies,[5] they are comparable with what has been reported

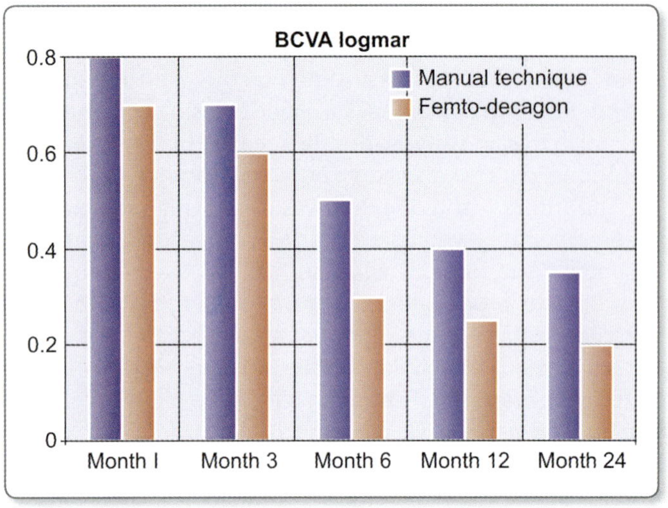

Fig. 4.8: Comparison postoperative best corrected visual acuity for PKP patients after manual and femtolaser trepanation
Abbreviation: PKP— penetrating keratoplasty

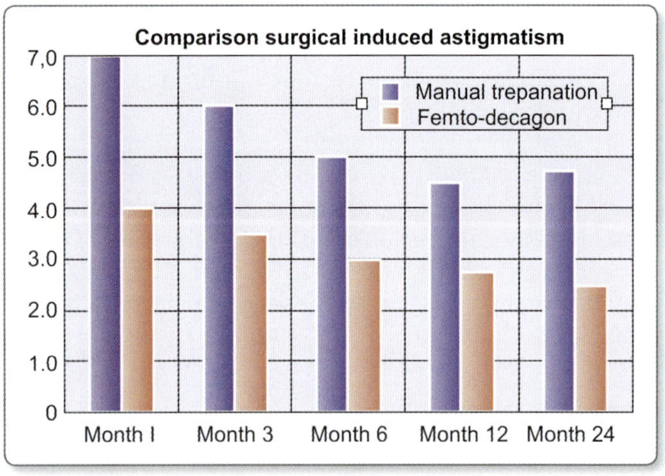

Fig. 4.9: Comparison of postoperative astigmatism for PKP patients after manual and femtolaser trepanation
Abbreviation: PKP— penetrating keratoplasty

for top hat and zig-zag femto-perforating keratoplasty, as well as studies that also use decagonal cuts. A study from Marseille reported similar results using decagonal corneas in 16 eyes.[6] The main difference in these published studies is the use of different femtosecond laser platforms—the Technolas femtosecond laser or the IntraLase femtosecond laser (Abbott Medical Optics, Santa Ana, CA) and then the sectional design.

The published studies where a femtosecond laser was used for corneal transplants have one thing in common—they all report exceptional cutting precision, rapid wound healing, the faster visual recovery and a higher effective clear optical zone but not always less induced astigmatism.

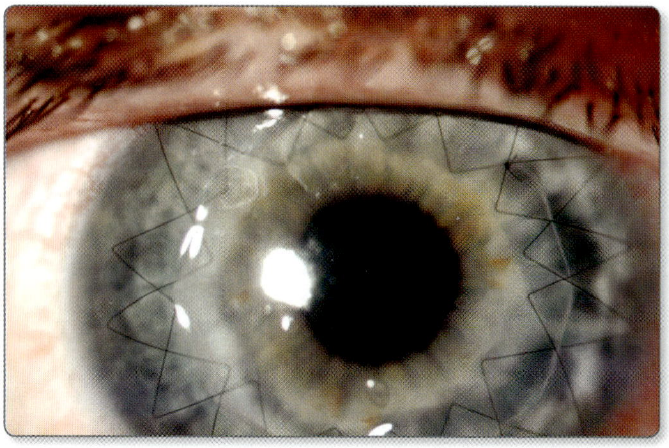

Fig. 4.10: Decagonal femto PKP 6 months postoperative view before suture removal
Abbreviation: PKP— penetrating keratoplasty

The key difference with the Technolas femtosecond laser compared to the IntraLase system is the patient interface that is used. With the IntraLase femtosecond laser, the interface completely flattens the cornea while with the Technolas system, corneal flattening and induced intraocular pressure is minimized due to the curved patient interface (Fig. 4.11).

In author's experience with the Technolas 520F, PKPs as well as DALKs are precise and the laser works well with transparent corneas, as well as cloudy or even scarred corneas. If the recipient cornea shows strong scars author tends to perform a double-pass femto cut—the first cut starts at 1,300 µm and stops at 150 µm under the corneal surface. The second pass starts again at 1,300 µm and ends in the patient interface +150 µm. This double-pass technique shows significant better results when removing scared recipient corneas (Figs 4.12A and B).

In these eyes, the corneas are well adapted, with no or only small corneal folds.

Overall, the use of the femtosecond laser allows for reduced suturing, excellent wound healing and stable anterior chambers.

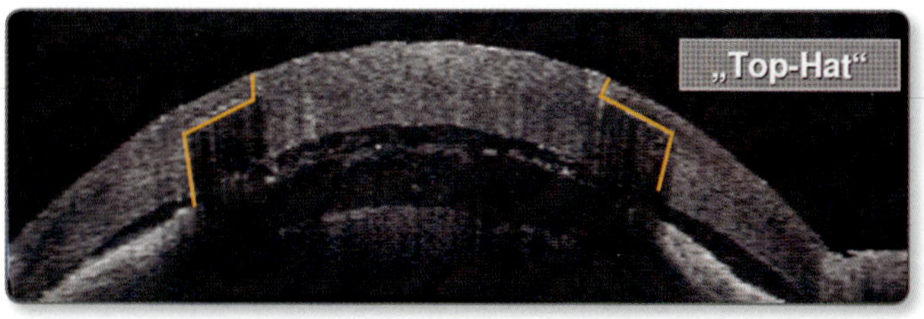

Fig. 4.11: Top-hat shaped penetrating keratoplasty

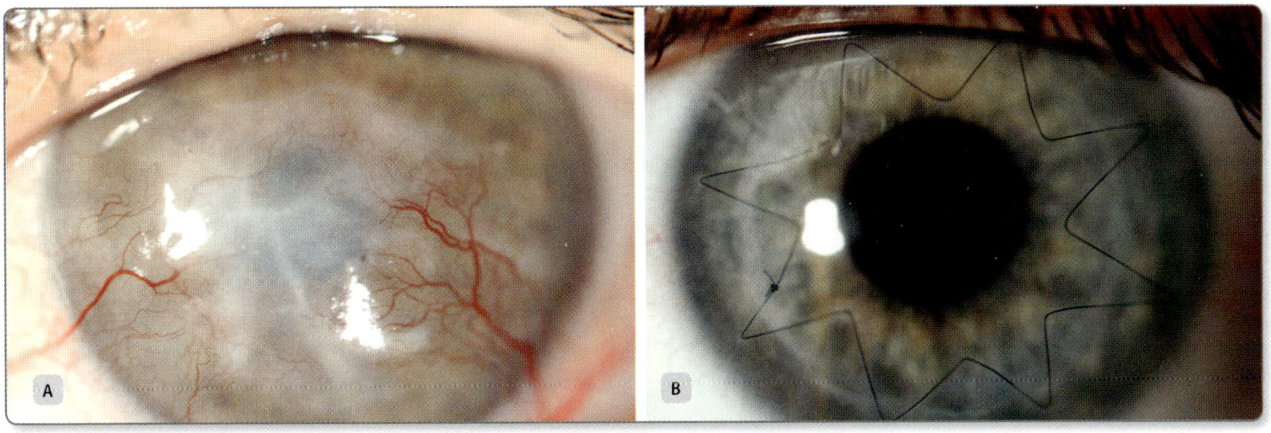

Figs 4.12A and B: Scared cornea (A) after crosslinking and then (B) at 6-month postoperative PKP (same eye!)
Abbreviation: PKP— penetrating keratoplasty

DEEP ANTERIOR LAMELLAR GRAFTS

As with PKP, the software on the Technolas femtosecond laser allows for full customization of deep anterior lamellar grafts procedures. This customization includes bed style, rim shape (circular, tophat and mushroom) and rim style (circular, orientation teeth, decagon). There is also an option for orientation markings to help facilitate graft placement.

With its precise depth and diameter selection, as well as a software predictor for anterior and posterior diameter, the pachymetry, particularly in keratoconic patients is very accurate, allowing you to enter the pachymetry data 1:1 into the software mask.

Compared with manual techniques, the procedure is faster and far more precise. This enables an operation that is as traumatic as possible (Fig. 4.13).

The use of deep anterior lamellar grafts, compared to PKP, reduces the risk of graft rejection, with faster wound healing and suture removal. The suture technique is the same as described above. In author's experience with the Technolas laser, even opaque tissue in the recipient eye can be dissected. The main difference that he has seen between this technique and PKP is related to residual astigmatism. It seems that keeping the integrity of the globe with DALK means that the astigmatic design remains almost untouched. This issue is a point that requires further evaluation.

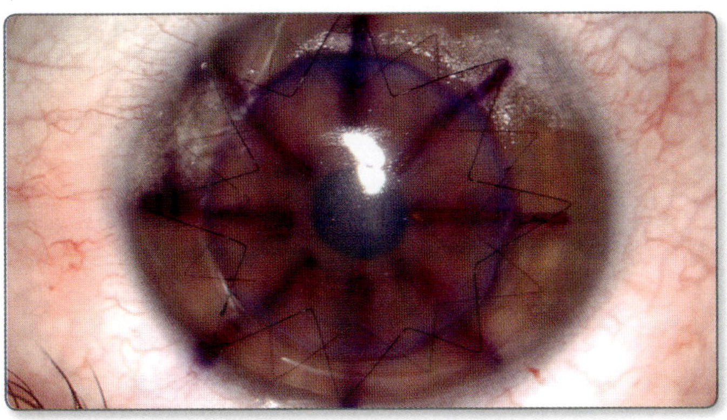

Fig. 4.13: Lamellar keratoplasty at the end of surgery, centered over the pupil and intrastromal air still remains at 10- and 2 o'clock

ENDOTHELIAL KERATOPLASTY/ POSTERIOR LAMELLAR GRAFTS

The most difficult form of corneal transplantation, the first successful posterior lamellar graft procedure using the Technolas femtosecond laser was performed by Dr Mark Tomalla, Duisburg, Germany, in November 2006. During endothelial keratoplasty, the patient's non-functioning cells are removed and replaced with healthy donor cells. The advantage to the procedure is that it is less traumatic than a PKP procedure, with a reduced risk of transplant rejection. However, the procedure was quite technically challenging until the advent of the femtosecond laser (Fig. 4.14). Precise shapes and depth can be achieved with the laser, with more predictable outcomes and a reduction in the manipulation of the cornea can be obtained when using this platform. A consistent ablation pattern ensures a smoother bed and easier extraction of endothelial cells.

The procedure is performed through a small incision, with the removal and replacement of the endothelium, followed by placement. An air bubble is then used to unfold the donor cells and position it against the recipient cornea. Typically, the donor tissue attaches to the recipient cornea, without sutures, within minutes of implantation.

The advantages of using the Technolas femtosecond laser in this procedure include the ability to obtain a precise

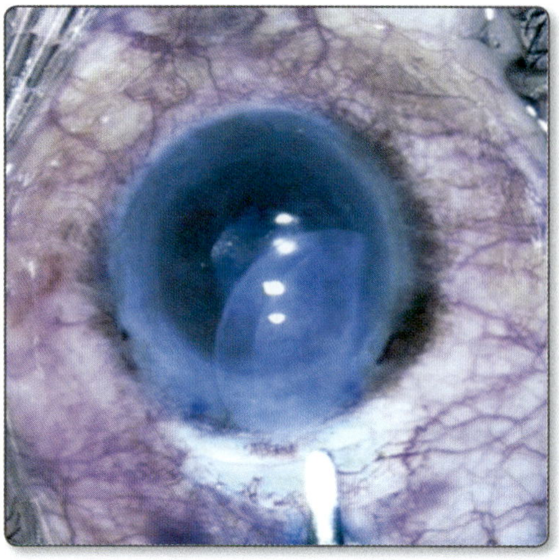

Fig. 4.14: Posterior endothelial graft being inserted through the incision prior to final positioning

cut that is 100–150 µm above Descemet's membrane, with a smoother bed and easier extraction of the endothelial cells. An added benefit is the reduced reliance on guesswork when performing this procedure.

ADDITIONAL PROCEDURES PERFORMED WITH THE TECHNOLAS FEMTOSECOND LASER

Custom Shape Astigmatic Keratotomies (AK)

This procedure is quick (± 10 seconds) and can correct up to 10 diopters of astigmatism, with a high degree of precision, with minimal risk of anterior chamber perforation. It works with all currently published AK nomograms.

The software is fully customizable, including adjustable visual orientation of the planning software, using these parameters:

- Radius
- Opening angles (alpha)
- Arc length
- Angle beta
- Depth (incisions both same or individual).

Custom Shape Implantable Corneal Ring Segments (ICRS)

Using the Custom Shape software, virtually every parameter in this procedure is customizable, including the inner diameter to obtain the required ring width, as well as the manufacturer recommended outer diameter. The software allows the surgeon to create one or two fully adjustable incisions—either cross cut or along the arc, while the cut depth is adjustable in 10-µm steps.

As with all corneal procedures performed on the Technolas femtosecond laser, surgeons have full visibility during the procedure and can use any type of corneal ring with the laser (Fig. 4.15).

COSTS

There is one disadvantage with femto keratoplasty, regardless of the manufacturer of the laser. It creates considerably higher costs than manual trephination and in this way is obviously not economical. While the costs for a good manual trephine system average 40,000 Euros, the cost of a femtosecond laser is about 500,000 Euros. Additionally, about 400 Euros per month is needed for rent of the room, as well as 30,000 Euros for the purchase of an air conditioning system. The annual medicotechnical inspection also costs approximately 30,000 Euros. There is even more: The cost per case, the so-called procedure fee', consumes another 300 Euros. If the femtosecond laser and the air conditioning system are financed over a period of 5 years, about 10,000 Euros/month are payable. Including annual inspection and rent of the room, this adds up to 13,500 Euros per month or 162,000 Euros per year. If a patient decides in favor of Femto keratoplasty following informed consent including benefits and risks, clarity with respect to the increased costs must be explained.

When you take into account the advantages—considerably quicker physical and visual rehabilitation, quicker ability to work and considerably less postoperative medical care and costs—the additional costs of about 2,000 Euros, with about 100 applications per year, can be recovered.

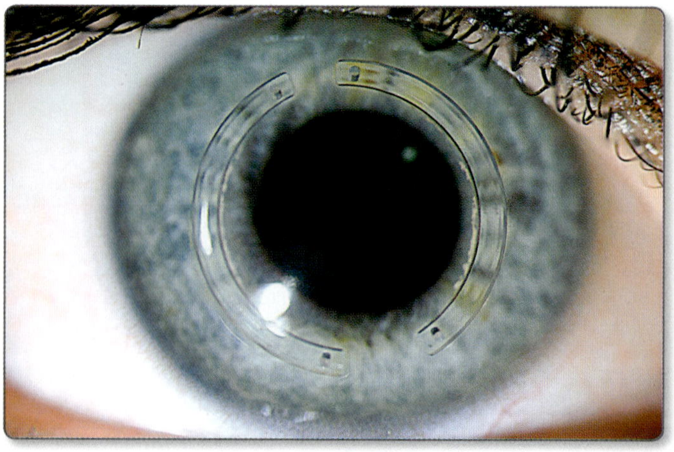

Fig. 4.15: Keraring segments at 12-month postoperative for treatment of keratoconus

In this way this new technology cannot only produce much more precise technical results than the human hand, but it may also reduce medical expenses. Even if this was not the case, Femto keratoplasty, according to the current state of knowledge, offers a further development for the benefit and well-being of the patients in all respects.

REFERENCES

1. Zirm E. Eine erfolgreiche totale Keratoplastik (A successful total keratoplasty) (1906). Refract Corneal Surg. 1989;5:258-61.
2. Seitz B. Aktueller Stand der perforierenden Keratoplastik. Klin Monatsbl Augenheilkd. 2010;227.
3. Barraquer JI. Two-Level keratoplasty. Int Ophthalmol Clin. 1963;3:515-39.
4. Busin M. A new lamellar wound configuration for penetrating keratoplasty surgery. Arch Opthalmol. 2003;121:260-5.
5. Price FW, Price MO. Femtosecond laser shaped penetrating keratoplasty: one-year results utilizing a top-hat configuration. Am J Ophthalmol. 2008;145:210-4.
6. Proust H, Baeteman C, Matonti F, et al. Femtosecond laser-assisted decagonal penetrating keratoplasty. Am J of Ophthalmol. 2011;151:29-34.

Chapter

5

Femtosecond Laser Corneal Applications: WaveLight FS200

Georg Gerten, Uwe Oberheide

CHAPTER OUTLINE

Technology Description

- All in one system: Femtosecond and excimer laser
- High pulse frequency of 200 kHz for femtosecond laser

Corneal Therapeutic Applications

- Capability in performing a combination of anterior and posterior annular, sagittal cuts as well as surface parallel lamellar cuts allowing nearly any shape of the transplanted tissue from anterior lamellar to posterior lamellar as well as penetrating keratoplasty
- Penetrating keratoplasty technique

TECHNOLOGY DESCRIPTION

The WaveLight FS200 femtosecond laser is the first femtosecond laser to be commercialized by Alcon Laboratories (Ft. Worth, TX). Combined with the WaveLight EX500 excimer laser, the two lasers create a refractive suite covering femtosecond flap preparation and refractive correction in a combined system (Figs 5.1A and B). Although flap creation is the most frequent use, the principles of photo disruption using infrared femtosecond laser pulses allow nearly any kind of three-dimensional corneal cuts and, therefore, therapeutic corneal applications.

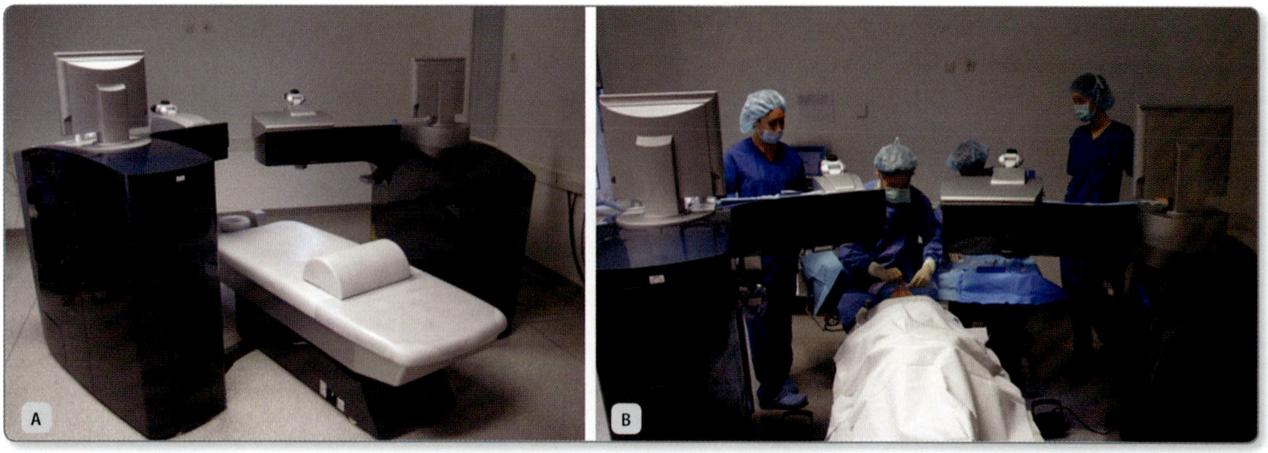

Figs 5.1A and B: WaveLight FS200

The WaveLight FS200 system is a near-infrared laser emitting laser pulses with a 350 fs pulse duration at 1,030 nm wavelength and 2.4 μJ maximum pulse energy. The high-pulse frequency of 200 kHz allows for fast treatments and very short applanation and vacuum times. For example, creation, of a 9 mm flap can be cut within 6 seconds, depending on the type of customizable spot/line separation and adjusted energy settings.[1]

A 2010 technical evaluation of the FS200 by Mrochen, et al found that features, such as optical design, pulse energy, and scanning algorithms "allow reproducibility for tissue cutting with a standard deviation of less than 10 μm in depth and 0.1 mm laterally". The report noted that increase in intraocular pressure of up to 150 mm Hg during applanation was in line with what had been previously reported with other femtosecond laser systems.[2]

An animal and cadaver eye study performed to evaluate the cut quality and cellular damage with this system was published in 2009 looked at the surface of the cornea, structure and ultrastructure of the corneal cells and stroma following flap creation.[3] Researchers used light microscopy (hematoxylin and eosin, periodic acid-Schiff and Picrosirius red staining), transmission electron microscopy and scanning electron microscopy (SEM) to perform the evaluation. The results showed that there were no side effects from the laser. In addition, the area around the flap cut was minimally affected, while the keratocytes and collagen fibers showed minimal changes. The SEM analysis showed smooth surfaces and precise side cuts. The same applies to cornea transplant surgery: absolutely smooth surfaces are one of the advantages of femtosecond laser cuts versus conventional manual trephination (Figs 5.2A and B).

A larger animal eye study, published in 2012 looked at the precision, morphology and histology in pig eyes using the WaveLight FS200 to cut corneal flaps in pig eyes.[4] Thirty-six pig eyes were put into three flap thickness groups: 100 μm, 130 μm or 180 μm. Additionally, flap diameters were varied from 8.0 mm to 9.5 mm. The completed flaps were measured with a micrometer gauge, as well as a sliding caliper. Flaps also underwent histologic examination.

The mean flap thickness 96.33 ± 7.45 μm (intended thickness: 100 μm), 134.67 ± 4.96 μm (intended thickness: 130 μm), and 174.59 ± 9.35 μm (intended thickness: 180 μm). The mean flap diameter was 8.03 ± 0.15 mm (intended diameter: 8.0 mm), 8.56 ± 0.10 mm (intended diameter: 8.5 mm) and 9.09 ± 0.10 mm (intended diameter: 9.0 mm), and 9.54 ± 0.15 mm (intended diameter: 9.5 mm). Histologic examination showed very little to almost no change in the structure of the corneal stroma.

CORNEAL THERAPEUTIC APPLICATIONS

Therapeutic applications of corneal cuts cover intrastromal corneal ring implantation as well as different types of keratoplasty procedures. For femtosecond penetrating keratoplasties (PKPs), the FS200 can be programed to perform a combination of anterior and posterior annular, sagittal cuts as well as surface parallel lamellar cuts allowing nearly any shape of the transplanted tissue from anterior lamellar to posterior lamellar as well as PKP.

When choosing PKP treatments, the height, diameter and angle to the surface normal of the cornea are entered

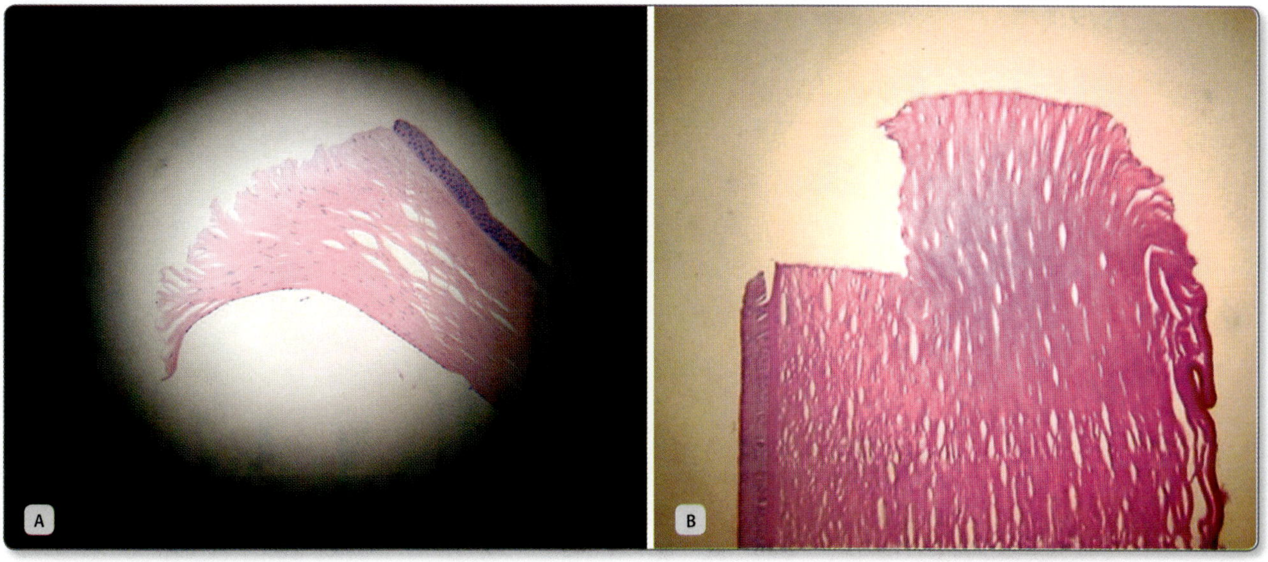

Figs 5.2A and B: (A) Corneal image obtained from femtosecond laser; (B) Conventional manual trephination of cornea

in the laser. Depending on these parameter settings the surface completes the pattern by connecting the endpoints of both cuts resulting in a surface parallel or tilted lamellar cut for most patterns.

These cuts can combine to shapes like mushroom, top-hat or zigzag pattern. Depending on the corneal pathology/anatomy, a corresponding laser pattern can be used. Example: In keratoconus, one goal is to achieve good visual acuity with a minimal risk of endothelial rejection. For transplantation in such a keratoconic cornea, a mushroom pattern could be appropriate (Figs 5.3A to D). This profile provides a large optical (epithelial) surface and minimizes endothelial diameter of the transplant.

In Fuchs´dystrophy maximum endothelial surface may be achieved by choosing a top-hat profile (Figs 5.4A and B). If corneal stability is of major concern, a barrel could be the pattern of choice (Figs 5.5A and B).

Due to the high pulse frequency of 200 kHz, a cutting time for a transplant with a mushroom shape of 8 mm anterior diameter and 1,200 µm depth (starting in the anterior chamber) can be achieved in approximately 45 seconds. In combination with the double-vacuum cones, which are first fixated to the eye and then the patient interface is fixed with a second vacuum between the suction ring and patient interface without mechanical fixation, the overall procedure time can be further reduced.

The advanced suction technology of the suction ring with peripheral spacers minimizes sclera deformation during suction and therefore keeps the intraocular pressure at a reasonable level.

The large diameter of the applanation glass allows for software adjustable laser pattern centration after suction is engaged without minimizing the diameter of the laser pattern over a wide range.

Furthermore, the beam-control-check technology of the wavelight FS200 measures each patient interface prior to surgery and adjusts any deviation to ensure a precise cutting depth within ± 5 µm to the intended cutting depth.

With all this technological background further corneal applications like arcuate incisions and corneal pockets for inlays that are not yet supported at the moment, will be implemented in the system soon.

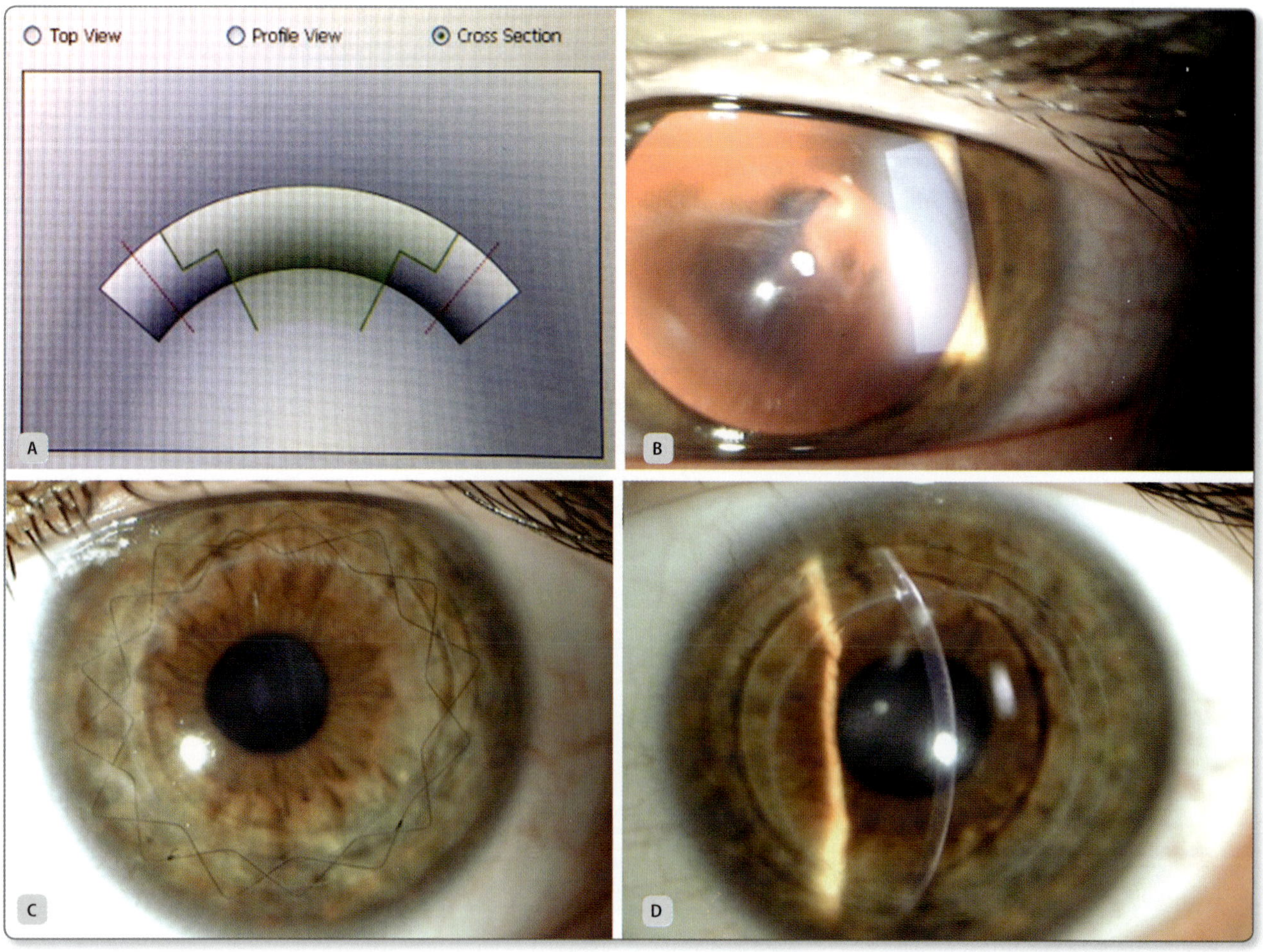

Figs 5.3A to D: Mushroom pattern in keratoconic corneal transplantation

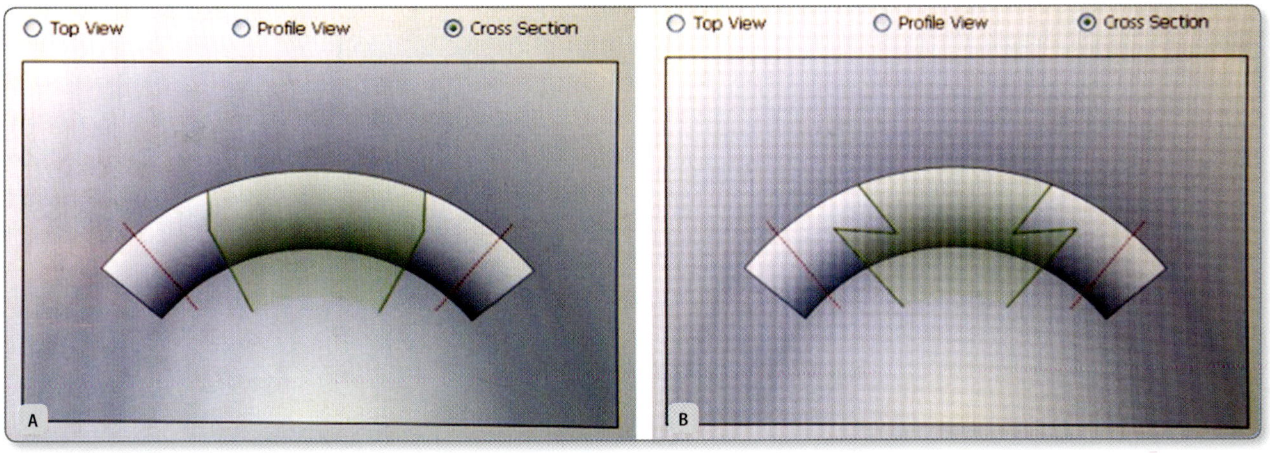

Figs 5.4A and B: Top-hat profile in Fuchs´dystrophy

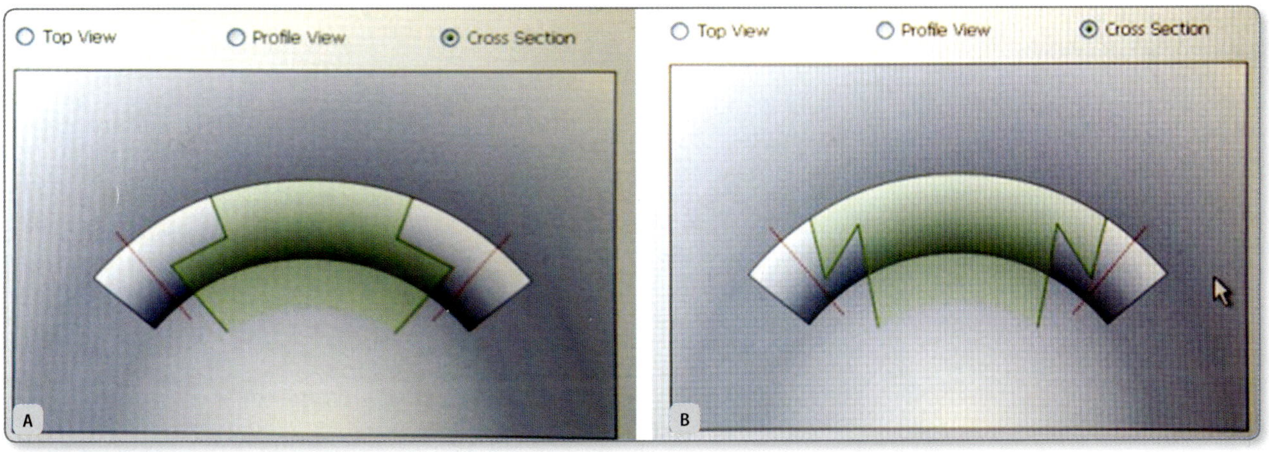

Figs 5.5A and B: Barrel shape

REFERENCES

1. Alcon laboratories. Company data on file.
2. Mrochen M, Wüllner C, Krause J, et al. Technical aspects of the WaveLight FS200 femtosecond Laser. J Refract Surg. 2010;26(10):S833-40.
3. Winkler von Mohrenfels C, Khoramnia R, Maier MM, et al. Cut quality of a new femtosecond laser system. (Article in German). Klin Monbl Augenheilkd. 2009;226(6):470-4.
4. Khoramnia R, Salgado JP, Lohmann CP, et al. Precision, morphology, and histology of corneal flap cuts using a 200-kHz femtosecond laser. Eur J Ophthalmol. 2012;22(2):161-7.

Chapter

6

Femtosecond Laser-Assisted Superficial Lamellar Keratectomy for the Treatment of Superficial Corneal Leukomas

Jorge L Alió, Felipe Soria, Alfredo Vega

CHAPTER OUTLINE

Preoperative Considerations

- Indications of corneal excision as an alternative to corneal graft surgery
- Ophthalmological examination
- General considerations concerning the indication

Understanding the Surgical Technique

- Calculation of the corneal depth for the excision procedure
- Smoothing of the stromal residual surface: Importance of the masking agent and fluorescein
- Evidence available
- Biomicroscopy
- Visual acuity
  - Refraction
  - Corneal topography and aberrometry
  - Complications

INTRODUCTION

Superficial corneal opacities following corneal dystrophies, infections and ocular trauma (including previous surgeries or refractive procedures) are a frequent cause of visual loss[1] and a frequent indication of corneal grafting. Despite the advances made in corneal transplantations still, immunological rejection[2-7] and a long visual recovery during the postoperative period[6-12] are the main issues in this procedure.

The authors published in the year 2004[13] the results of automated superficial lamellar keratectomy augmented by excimer Laser masked phototherapeutic keratectomy (PTK) in the management of severe superficial corneal opacities demonstrating that this procedure induces a significant improvement in corneal transparency and visual acuity in cases of corneal opacity caused by previous refractive surgery, ocular trauma and keratitis. Another authors have published that corneal scars may also be excised without grafting by lamellar keratectomy.[14,15]

In the era of femtosecond laser the combination with excimer laser gives us another possibility of treatment with the premise in trying to avoid corneal grafting: femtosecond laser-assisted superficial lamellar keratectomy.

In the year 2011, the authors published the results of femtosecond laser-assisted superficial lamellar keratectomy for the treatment of corneal leukomas,[16] showing that superficial corneal excision with femtosecond laser augmented with PTK laser smoothening assisted with 0.25% sodium hyaluronate improved visual acuity and could be considered as an alternative to more invasive procedures in patients with severe opacities. Moreover, the use of masking agents such as 0.25% sodium hyaluronate has been proposed in one of our previous studies. Using this masking agent can induce a significant improvement in corneal transparency and visual acuity of patients with corneal opacities.[17-20]

In the following chapter, the authors will describe the procedure and outcomes of superficial lamellar keratectomy aided with femtosecond laser technology and masked PTK as an alternative to corneal grafting.

PREOPERATIVE CONSIDERATIONS

Indications

- Superficial corneal scars (below 300 µm) (Fig. 6.1) with absence of new vessels because of the lack of capability of the femtosecond laser energy to cut vessels or to penetrate through vascularized tissues.
  - Infection: Must be inactive
  - Trauma: Includes surgical trauma [photorefractive keratectomy (PRK), Laser in-situ keratomileusis (LASIK), Pterygium]
  - Corneal dystrophies
- Stabilized refraction.

Ophthalmological examination should include:

- Topography (Fig. 6.2)
  - It is a mandatory study for the surgery, because will determine our possible visual outcomes.
- Pachymetry
  - Anterior optical coherence tomography (OCT): It is a mandatory preoperative study. Measuring the depth and longitude of the corneal scarring will allow us to determine the parameters our surgical planning (Figs 6.3A and B).

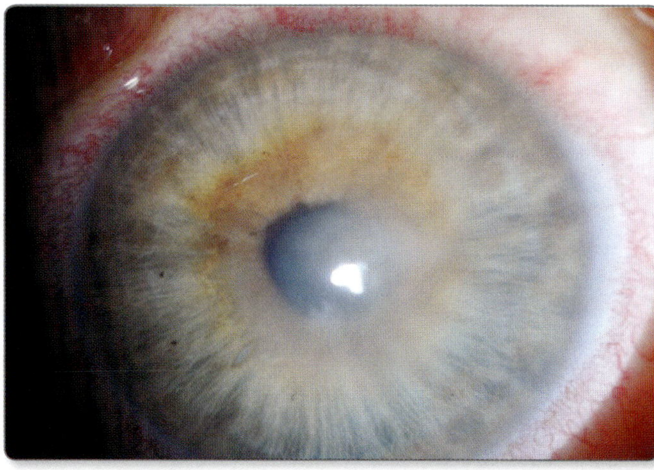

Fig. 6.1: Showing a superficial central leukoma

Preoperative Studies

A complete ophthalmological evaluation has to be made, having the absolute certainty of the potential vision of the patient. The surgeon must explain to the patient the expectations in terms of visual acuity that the patient will

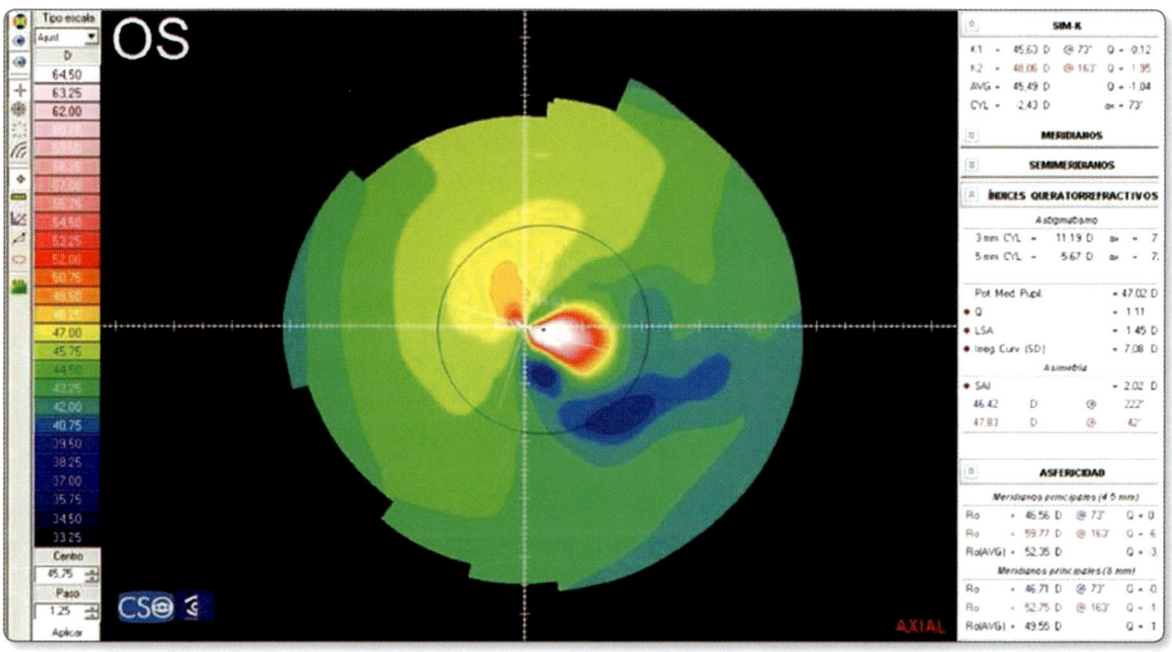

Fig. 6.2: Corneal topography of a central leukoma

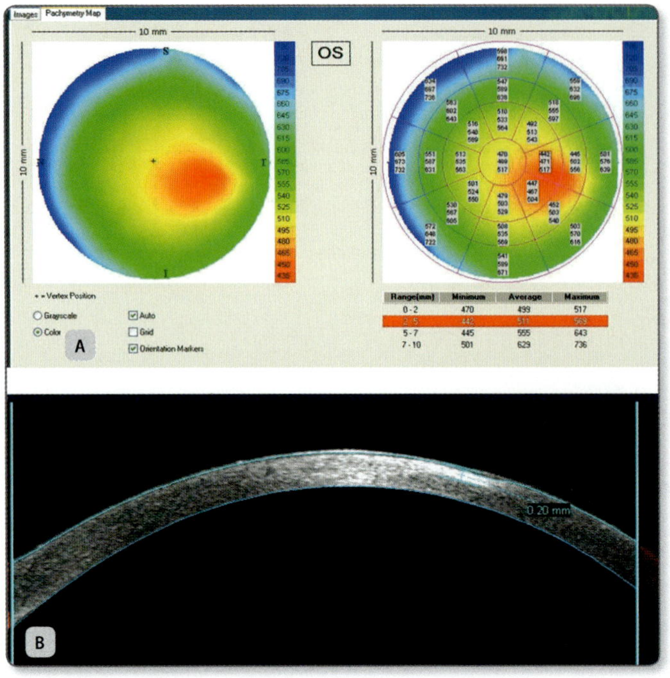

Figs 6.3A and B: Pachymetry and OCT of the same patient from previous images showing the depth and localization of the leukoma

achieve after the surgery and also to take in consideration that the final visual acuity will be achieved after 1 year.

General Considerations

Topical anesthesia is used during the whole procedure.

SURGICAL TECHNIQUE

A two-step surgical technique includes:

1. The first step consists in creating a free corneal cap using the femtosecond Laser. Like a rule of thumb the energy used in this procedure must double the amount of corneal refractive procedures because we are aiming to guarantee corneal dissection in the presence of opacities. The corneal cap thickness is selected according to the depth measured by OCT and a superior 4 mm hinge is created. Table 6.1 shows the parameter for flap creation.
2. The second step consists in the excimer laser ablation. Before activating the laser, a free cap is created, removing it with a crescent blade and a drop of 0.25% of sodium hyaluronate is instilled.

An ablation of 30–50 µm in a 6 mm area using PTK mode is programed. In our experiences, the ablation is done with the AMARIS excimer laser (SCHWIND eye-tech solutions GmbH & Co., Kleinostheim, Germany). A drop of fluorescein is instilled on the cornea; this is to monitor the disappearance of the masking agent. The absence of fluorescein indicates the complete removal of the viscoelastic masking solution.

As soon as the ablation is finished, mitomycin C 0.02% is applied for 1 minute following an intense washing with balanced salt solution. Finally, a bandage contact lens is placed.

Table 6.1: Flap creation parameter

Method	*Raster*
Diameter	9.0
Depth	This is the depth of the corneal scarring
Hinge	Superior
Hinge angle	45°
Bed energy	1.05
Spot sep	8
Line sep	8
Side cut energy	1.15
Side cut angle	70
Pocket enable	On
Pocket width	0.250
Pocket start depth	250
Pocket tang spot sep	5
Pocket rad spot sep	5

OUTCOMES[16]

Preserving the cornea of our patient is of tremendous importance, thus trying to avoid a corneal grafting is necessary when we face a superficial corneal leukoma.

The following study analyzed the visual outcomes of keratectomy assisted by femtosecond Laser. Twelve eyes (9 patients: 6 men and 3 women) with mean age of 46.1 ± 17.8 years (range, 21–71 years), various degrees of superficial corneal opacities, and the absence of corneal new vessels were included in this study. Table 6.2 shows the grade and maximal depth of the opacity in each case and Table 6.3 shows corneal haze-grading system.

Visual Acuity

The mean uncorrected visual acuity (UCVA) and best spectacle-corrected visual acuity (BSCVA) at the preoperative visit and at 1, 6 and 12 months are shown in Tables 6.4 and 6.5, respectively. Figure 6.4 shows the evolution of UCVA and BSCVA.

Table 6.2: Grade and maximal depth of the opacity in each case

Eye	*Cause of severe corneal scarring and opacity*	*Depth of opacity as measured by confocal microscope (mm)*	*Haze grade*
1	Corneal refractive (PRK)	195	3
2	Corneal refractive surgery (PRK)	201	3
3	Corneal dystrophy	170	4
4	Corneal dystrophy	195	4
5	Infectious keratitis	217	4
6	Corneal refractive surgery (RK followed by LASIK)	218	4
7	Pterygium surgery	298	3
8	Pterygium surgery	190	4
9	Corneal refractive surgery (complicated LASIK)	120	4
10	Corneal refractive surgery (PRK over a previous LASIK)	219	4
11	Corneal refractive surgery (PRK over a previous LASIK)	275	4
12	Corneal refractive surgery (PRK)	245	3

LASIK, laser assisted in situ keratomileusis; PRK, photorefractive keratectomy; RK, radial keratotomy

Table 6.3: Corneal haze-grading system

Grade	*Description*
0	Totally clear
0.5	Trace or faint corneal haze seen only by indirect broad tangential illumination
1	Haze of minimal density seen with difficulty with direct and diffuse illumination
2	Mild haze easily visible with direct focal slit illumination
3	Moderately dense opacity that partially obscures the iris details
4	Severely dense opacity that completely obscures the details of intraocular structures

Fantes FE, Hanna KD, Waring GO III, et al. Wound healing after excimer Laser keratomileusis (photorefractive keratectomy) in monkeys. Arch Ophthalmol. 1990;108:665-75.

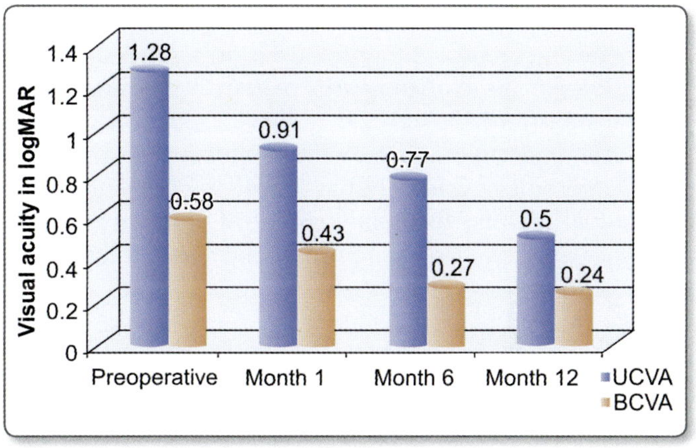

Fig. 6.4: Bar graph showing the evolution of UCVA and BSCVA preoperatively at 1, 6 and 12 months

Refraction

The sphere and cylinder mean values at the preoperative visit and at 1, 6 and 12 months postoperative are shown in Table 6.4.

Corneal Haze and Opacity

The causes of haze and scarring are listed in Table 6.2. The mean haze grade is 3.67 ± 0.49 (range, 3–4). The mean preoperative leukoma depth obtained by confocal

Table 6.4: The sphere and cylinder mean values at the preoperative visit and at 1, 6 and 12 months postoperative

	Sphere		*Cylinder*	
	Mean	*Range*	*Mean*	*Range*
Preoperative	−1.98 ± 5.05	−5.5 to +13	−1.35 ± 1.53	−5 to 0
Month 1	−0.25 ± 3.31	−6 to +6	−2.15 ± 1.60	−4 to 0
Month 6	+0.83 ± 3.04	−4.0 to 5.5	−2.44 ± 1.59	−4.5 to −0.75
Month 12	−0.25 ± 2.07	−4.75 to 1.75	−2.41 ± 1.36	−3.75 to −1

microscopy was 171.55 ± 55.58 mm. At the end of the study, none of the eyes had corneal haze as re-examined under the slit lamp using the haze-grading system (Table 6.5).

Corneal Topography and Aberrometry

Table 6.6 shows the preoperative and postoperative Sim K values, total aberration, astigmatism, higher-order aberration (HOA), and spherical-like and coma-like aberrations expressed as root-mean-square (RMS). As shown, we did not observe significant changes or progression in the topographic and aberrometric indexes analyzed for this study.

COMPLICATIONS

None of the eyes showed any complication during the postoperative follow-up of the study.

CONCLUSION

Encountering superficial corneal leukomas in our clinical practice is a common situation. Offering a procedure that will conserve the cornea of our patient is of tremendous clinical importance.

Automated superficial lamellar keratectomy augmented with hyaluronic-assisted PTK has proved to be an alternative to corneal grafting for management of severe superficial corneal opacity. Using femtosecond technology has allowed ophthalmic surgeons to perform a variety of corneal refractive procedures with high precision, offering numerous advantages over mechanical microkeratome devices in terms of visual quality, reproducibility and safety.[21] It is likely that a more regular and precise corneal excision was obtained with the use of the femtosecond Laser. The use of viscous masking agents increases the efficiency of the procedure by protecting the valleys in between peaks and leaving these peaks of pathology exposed to Laser treatment.[20] Using hyaluronate eyedrops also accelerates epithelial wound closure.[22,23] This procedure can improve visual acuity and optical quality vision of patients with superficial corneal opacities. A final comment that deserves the attention is that, although the good results in terms of BSCVA in majority of the patients, this was achieved between 6 months and 12 months.[16] Femtosecond Laser-assisted superficial lamellar keratectomy for the treatment of superficial corneal leukomas is an excellent alternative to more invasive procedures.

Table 6.5: Degree of haze at the preoperative visit and 12 months after surgery

	Degree of haze, n (%)				
	0	*I*	*II*	*III*	*IV*
Preoperative	–	–	–	4 (33)	8 (67)
Month 12	12 (100)	–	–	–	–

Table 6.6: Corneal topographic and aberrometric data

	Preoperative	Postoperative	P (CI = 95%)
K1	39.59 ± 6.36	39.13 ± 5.35	0.73 (NS)
K2	43.15 ± 4.29	42.20 ± 6.57	0.58 (NS)
Cylinder	3.55 ± 3.08	3.05 ± 2.47	0.28 (NS)
Total aberation RMS	7.81 ± 4.73	5.15 ± 1.40	0.26 (NS)
Astigmatism RMS	3.28 ± 3.88	2.38 ± 1.56	0.533 (NSS)
HOA RMS	4.54 ± 3.08	4.33 ± 4.79	0.85 (NS)
Spherical-like RMS	0.84 ± 0.47	0.95 ± 0.65	0.67 (NS)
Coma-like RMS	1.95 ± 0.98	1.48 ± 0.78	0.28 (NS)

NS, no significant difference; SS, statistically significant difference

REFERENCES

1. Whitcher JP, Srinivasan M, Upadhyay MP. Corneal blindness: a global perspective. Bull World Health Organ. 2001;79:214-21.
2. Biswas S, Suresh P, Bonshek RE, et al. Graft failure in human donor corneas due to transmission of herpes simplex virus. Br J Ophthalmol. 2000;84:701-5.
3. Naacke HG, Borderie VM, Bourcier T, et al. Outcome of corneal transplantation rejection. Cornea. 2001;20:350-3.
4. Lee HM, Naor J, Alhindi R, et al. Detection of hepatitis C virus in the corneas of seropositive donors. Cornea. 2001;20:37-40.
5. Jonas JB, Rank RM, Budde WM. Immunologic graft reactions after allogenic penetrating keratoplasty. Am J Ophthalmol. 2002;133:437-43.
6. Reinhard T, Böhringer D, Hüschen D, et al. Chronic endothelial cell loss of the graft after penetrating keratoplasty: influence of endothelial cell migration from graft to host. Klin Monbl Augenheilkd. 2002;219:410-6.
7. Reinhard T, Bocking A, Sundmacher R. Chronic endophthalmitis mimicking an endothelial immune reaction after penetrating keratoplasty. J Cataract Refract Surg. 2002;28:1475-7.
8. Rumelt S, Bersudsky V, Blum-Hareuveni T, et al. Preexisting and postoperative glaucoma in repeated corneal transplantation. Cornea. 2002;21:759-65.
9. McDonnell PJ, Falcon MG. The lamellar corneal graft for optical indications. Eye (Lond). 1988;2:390-4.
10. Shimazaki J. The evolution of lamellar keratoplasty. Curr Opin Ophthalmol. 2000;11:217-23.
11. Xie L, Shi W, Liu Z, et al. Lamellar keratoplasty for the treatment of fungal keratitis. Cornea. 2002;21:33-7.
12. Melles GR, Remeijer L, Geerards AJ, et al. A quick surgical technique for deep, anterior lamellar keratoplasty using visco-dissection. Cornea. 2000;19:427-32.
13. Alió JL, Javaloy J, Merayo J, et al. Automated superficial lamellar keratectomy augmented by excimer laser masked

PTK in the management of severe superficial corneal opacities. Br J Ophthalmol. 2004;88:1289-94.
14. Rasheed K, Rabinowitz Y. Superficial lamellar keratectomy using an automated microkeratome to excise corneal scarring caused by photorefractive keratectomy. J Cataract Refract Surg. 1999;25:1184-7.
15. Hafezi F, Mrochen M, Seiler T, et al. Anterior lamellar keratoplasty with a microkeratome: a method for managing complications after refractive surgery. J Refract Surg. 2003;19:52-7.
16. Alió JL, Agdeppa MC, Uceda-Montanes A. Femtosecond laser-assisted superficial lamellar keratectomy for the treatment of superficial corneal leukomas. Cornea. 2011;30:301-7.
17. Alio´ JL, Artola A, Claramente PJ, et al. Complications of photorefractive keratectomy for myopia: two year follow-up of 3,000 cases. J Cataract Refract Surg. 1998;24:619-26.
18. Alió JL, Belda JI, Shalaby AM. Correction of irregular astigmatism with excimer laser assisted by sodium hyaluronate. Ophthalmology. 2001;108:1246-60.
19. Kornmehl EW, Steinert RF, Puliafito CA. A comparative study of masking fluids for excimer laser phototherapeutic keratectomy. Arch Ophthalmol. 1991;109:860-3.
20. Fitzsimmons TD, Fagerholm P. Superficial keratectomy with 193 nm excimer laser: a reproducible model of corneal surface irregularities. Acta Ophthalmol (Copenh). 1991;69:641-4.
21. Soong HK, Malta JB. Femtosecond lasers in ophthalmology. Am J Ophthalmol. 2009;147:189-97.
22. Nishida T, Nakamura M, Mishima H, et al. Hyaluronan stimulates corneal epithelial migration. Exp Eye Res. 1991;53:753-8.
23. Sugiyama T, Miyauchi S, Machida A, et al. The effect of sodium hyaluronate on the migration of rabbit corneal epithelium. II. The effect of topical administration. J Ocul Pharmacol. 1991;7:53-64.

Chapter

7

Artificial Anterior Chamber Systems Used for Femtosecond Laser Corneal Graft Surgery

Juan Álvarez de Toledo, Rafael I Barraquer-Compte, María F de la Paz

CHAPTER OUTLINE

- Relevance of the artificial anterior chamber for the transition to femtosecond corneal grafting surgery
- Description of the most relevant available artificial anterior chamber models
  - Non-disposable artificial anterior chambers
  - Disposable artificial anterior chambers
- How to use an artificial anterior chamber in femtosecond laser-assisted keratoplasty
- Complications and hot to avoid them
- Specific practical recommendations
  - Ensure that the donor corneoscleral button has a wide rim
  - Check for adequate pressure inside the artificial anterior chamber, avoid any collapse
  - Proper centering of the cutting pattern in the corneal tissue

INTRODUCTION

The use of an artificial anterior chamber (AAC) is a mandatory step to obtain the donor tissue during the surgical procedure of femto-keratoplasty.[1] All femtosecond lasers work very precisely to perform the corneal tissue cutting, but a stable and fixed contact with the tissue to achieve this high precision is needed. When performing femtosecond laser surgery in a human eye, a suction device is fixed to the eyeball. This suction device can be incorporated inside the cone of the laser or can be independent, as a suction ring, which is fixed first to the eye and later to the laser cone. In any case, a suction mechanism is needed to stabilize the tissue against the planar or curved surface of the laser cone.

When we are planning to perform a femtosecond laser cut in a donor cornea, the donor tissue can be obtained from the eye bank as a fresh whole eyeball or as a corneoscleral button. If we obtain a complete eyeball, then the procedure of cutting with the femtosecond laser is similar to that in the human recipient, using the suction device. Usually, donor fresh eyeballs have a low intraocular pressure and achieving a good suction is very difficult, making this option not recommended and discarded by most of the experts.

Nowadays, the majority of the eye banks work with liquid storage media to preserve the corneal tissue and only a corneoscleral button can be obtained. The use of an AAC is then mandatory to manipulate this type of tissue. The recent growth of other corneal lamellar surgical procedures,[2,3] such as Descemet's stripping endothelial keratoplasty (DSEK), Descemet's stripping automated endothelial keratoplasty (DSAEK) and Deep anterior lamellar keratoplasty (DALK) have increased the demand of tissue to be processed in an AAC, and different models of disposable and non-disposable devices have been introduced in the market. When donor tissue is to be utilized in an AAC, the diameter of the corneoscleral button should be larger to be properly held in the device, such that the diameter of the tissue prepared in the eye banks has shifted in the recent years from 14 mm to 16–17 mm.

When we use an AAC mounted corneoscleral button for femtosecond laser cutting, there is no need to apply the suction mechanism or the suction ring adapted to the laser, but it is very important to keep an adequate pressure inside the chamber to achieve a precise cut of the donor. In this chapter, authors have described the different models of AAC available and their use in femto-keratoplasty.

DESCRIPTION OF ARTIFICIAL ANTERIOR CHAMBERS MODELS

There are basically two types of AACs we can use: Disposable and non-disposable.

Non-disposable Artificial Anterior Chambers

Because of the increase of corneal lamellar procedures, non-disposable AAC have been widely used to perform the donor cutting or dissection like in superficial anterior lamellar keratoplasty (SALK), DALK, DSEK or DSAEK. They are made of reusable stainless steel and were mainly designed to perform SALK or DSAEK procedures. The most popular is the Moria AAC (Fig. 7.1), designed initially for anterior lamellar therapeutic keratoplasty (ALTK) but used at present to perform the microkeratome assisted endothelial keratoplasty (DSAEK). Other microkeratome manufacturers as Gebauer or Ziemer have designed their own nonreusable AACs (Fig. 7.2), also for DSAEK procedures. All of them can be used to prepare the corneal tissue with the femtosecond laser systems.

In the Moria AAC, the corneoscleral disk is gently mounted while a continuously irrigating balanced salt solution (BSS) solution is connected to the silicone tube. The stream of the solution is stopped when the disk is completely placed. This maneuver avoids the presence of air bubbles inside the anterior chamber. Then the locker ring is positioned (Fig. 7.3) and the elevating screw is rotated (Fig. 7.4) to firmly lock the tissue against it. Pressure can be measured with a Barraquer tonometer (Fig. 7.5) to ensure the appropriate level. Also pachymetry of the corneal tissue can be performed at this time (Fig. 7.6). The tissue is then already prepared to be cut with the femtosecond laser.

In all models, there are one or two ports with silicone tubing. Once the corneoscleral button is mounted and

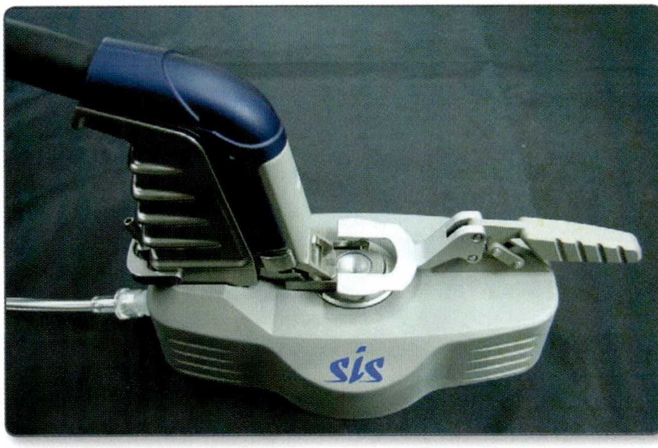

Fig. 7.2: Ziemer´s artificial anterior chamber is designed to be used with the AMADEUS II microkeratome. It can be used also for femto-keratoplasty if laser cone can fit through the locking mechanism

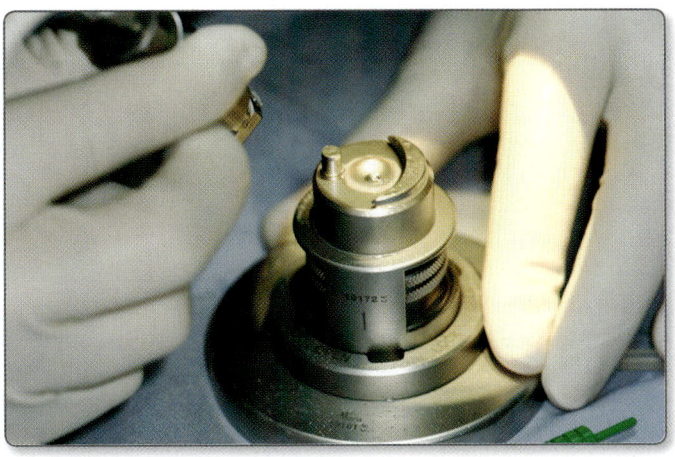

Fig. 7.1: Moria's anterior lamellar therapeutic keratoplasty (ALTK) artificial anterior chamber (AAC) holding the corneoscleral button. This device is routinely used to perform Descemet's stripping automated endothelial keratoplasty (DSAEK) procedures but can also be utilized in femto-keratoplasty

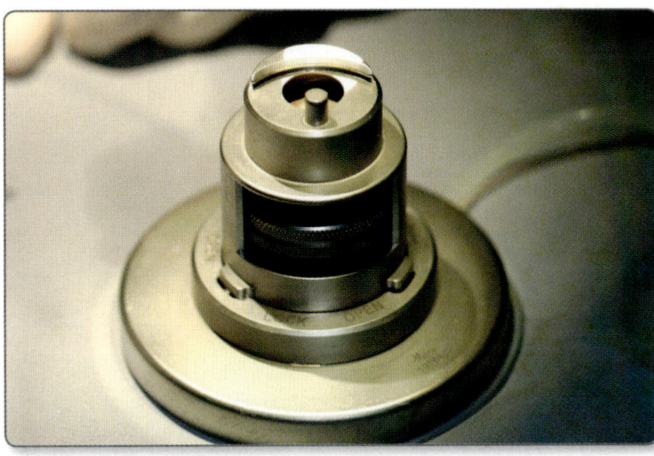

Fig. 7.3: Locker ring of the Moria´s artificial anterior chamber set in position with the tissue mounted in the elevating screw set in the down position

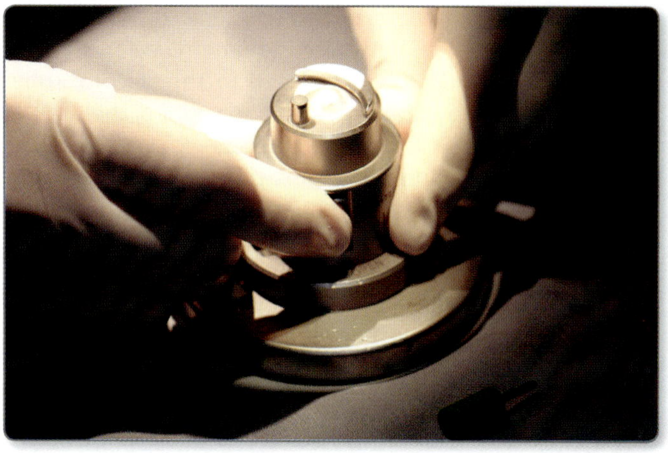

Fig. 7.4: Rotating the elevation screw to firmly lock the tissue and seal the artificial anterior chamber

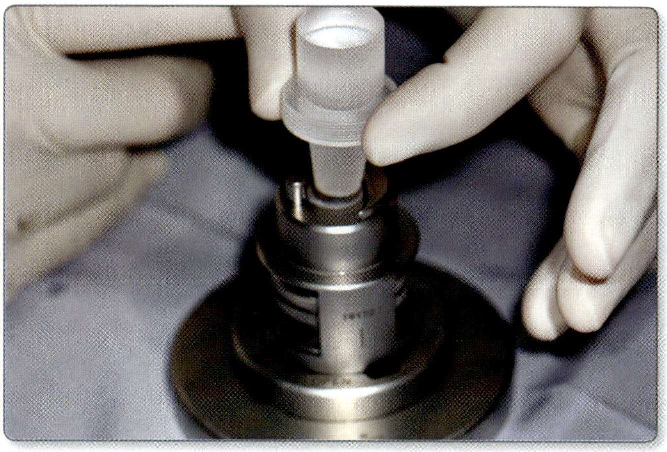

Fig. 7.5: Barraquer´s tonometer is used to properly measure an adequate pressure inside the artificial anterior chamber

locked in position, the adequate pressure inside the anterior chamber is achieved connecting a BSS solution bottle at a height between 80 cm to 120 cm. Maintaining this pressure inside the anterior chamber is very important in femtosecond laser cutting of the corneal tissue. If the pressure is too low, an excess of fluid can be seen in the borders of the applanation area. This can interfere with the precision of the cut; also, most femtosecond lasers require a minimum contact pressure to enable the system to activate the laser beam. If the pressure is too high, the contact area between the laser cone and the tissue will be usually smaller than the programed cutting diameter. Slight adjustments of the pressure inside the AAC, once there is contact between the laser cone and the tissue, may be necessary before starting the cut. This is to find the adequate value to allow the laser system to fire and obtain an adequate contact diameter (Fig. 7.7).

Disposable Artificial Anterior Chambers

The use of disposable AACs has spread worldwide because of its technical simplicity and to meet the legal regulations in the manipulation of human tissue. Single use instrumentation is another step to minimize the chance of contamination and transmission of severe infectious diseases,[4] such as AIDS, viral hepatitis or prion-related diseases, when donor tissue needs to be processed.

There are several disposable devices in the market: the Barron disposable AAC, the Moria disposable AAC and the Coronet disposable AAC.

Coronet Disposable Artificial Anterior Chambers (Figs 7.8 and 7.9)

The Coronet AAC (Network Medical Products Ltd. UK) is unique in concept in that one-chamber fits all sizes of donor graft.

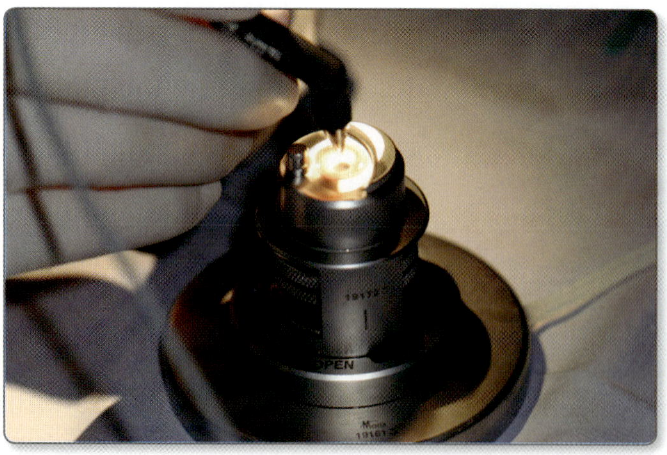

Fig. 7.6: Ultrasound pachymetry can be easily performed to measure corneal thickness in any point. It is critical in planning the femtosecond cutting parameters, especially in lamellar procedures

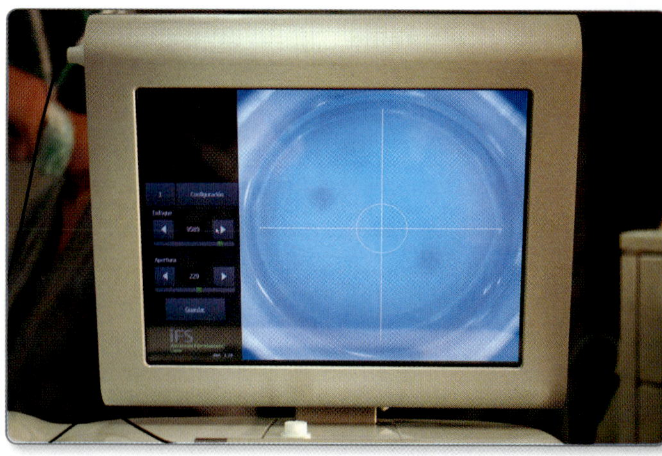

Fig. 7.7: Checking of the applanation area through the screen of the laser system

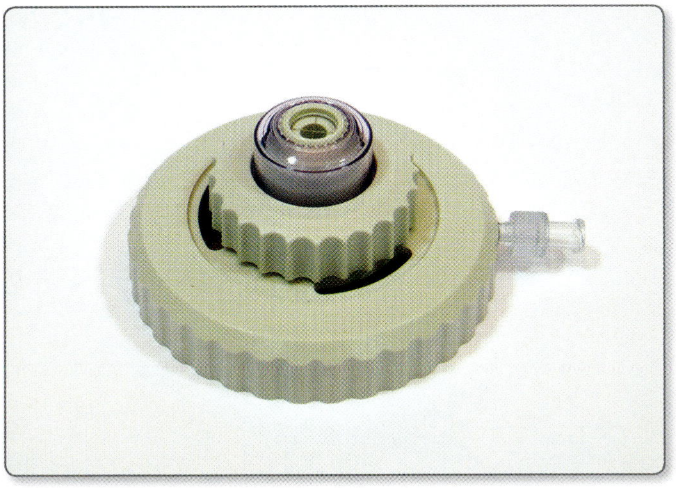

Fig. 7.8: Coronet artificial anterior chamber assembled

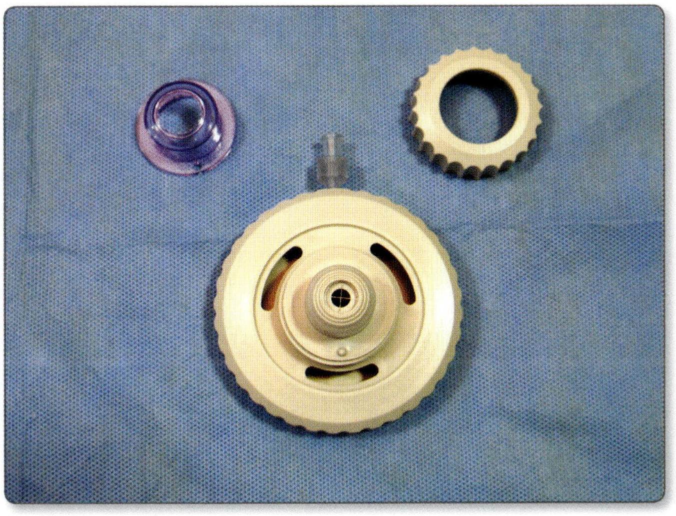

Fig. 7.9: Coronet artificial anterior chamber disassembled with its three pieces. It has a base with one irrigating port, a tissue retainer and a locking ring

The chamber is suitable for any size donor graft tissue from 14.5 mm to 18 mm. For this purpose, two tissue retaining heads are supplied with the chamber: a small retainer to accommodate graft tissue from 14.5 mm to 16 mm and a large retainer to accommodate graft tissue from 17 mm to 18 mm. The tissue is clamped into position on the top of the pedestal by the tissue retainer, which grips the tissue gently around the scleral ring and seals the chamber. It also has a cross line in the base to adequately center the corneal tissue. It has one port that fits standard Luer connections.

Moria Disposable Artificial Anterior Chambers (Figs 7.10 and 7.11)

This disposable anterior chamber has been recently designed by Moria SA in France to perform the ultrathin method of donor cutting for DSAEK. It consists of a plastic base, a metal chamber cover and a white plastic screw that locks the tissue in position. There are two Luer ports with two one-way stopcocks. For the ultrathin technique of cutting, a dovetail is also included, but it is not needed in femtosecond laser cutting. Its design allows simple use with all the femtosecond lasers cones.

Barron Disposable Artificial Anterior Chambers (Fig. 7.12)

This device is the most utilized AAC around the world to prepare the corneal donor. This disposable AAC (Katena Products Inc., NJ, USA) is composed of three pieces—base with tissue pedestal, tissue retainer and locking ring. The base has two ports with silicone tubing—in-line pinch clamps and female Luer connectors. Either port may be used to inject or aspirate viscoelastic material, BSS, preservation

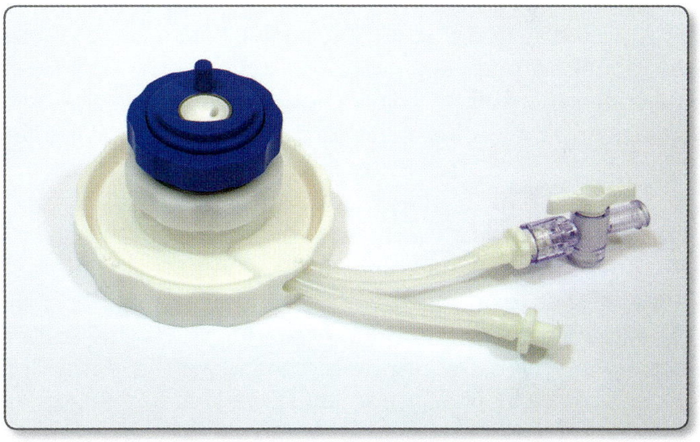

Fig. 7.10: Moria´s disposable artificial anterior chamber assembled

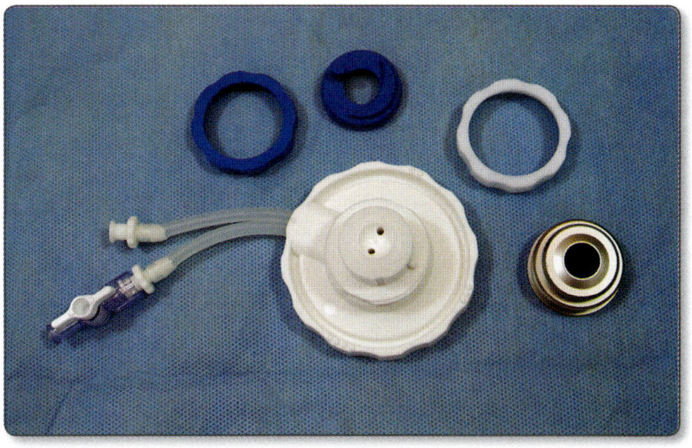

Fig. 7.11: Moria´s artificial anterior chamber disassembled in its four pieces: the base with two irrigating ports, a tissue retainer, a locking ring and a microkeratome adapter ring to perform the UltraThin technique in Descemet's stripping automated endothelial keratoplasty (DSAEK) procedures

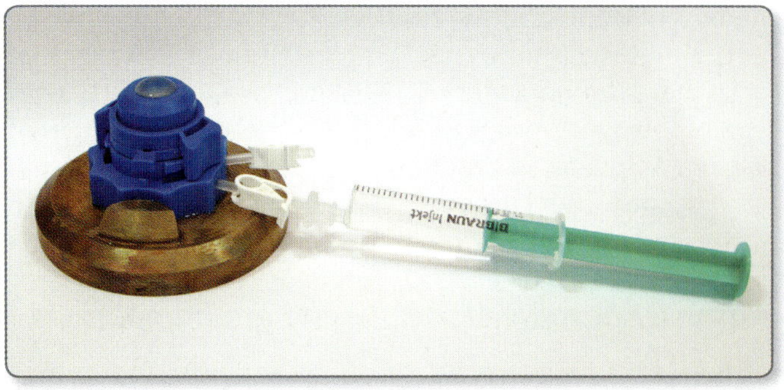

Fig. 7.12: Barron´s artificial anterior chamber assembled and mounted onto a custom made metal base to ease the handling of the chamber and ensure its stability

media, or air. After the donor corneoscleral button is placed onto the base, the tissue retainer is then carefully placed over the unit with the guideposts aligned; then, the tissue retainer is advanced to the bottom of the base. The AAC is then secured by placing the locking ring over the unit and turning it until the locked position is reached. Once the donor corneoscleral button is sealed onto the AAC, the surgeon is able to adjust the pressure within the unit by injecting the desired solution through the two available ports. The Barron AAC is designed in a bright blue color to provide a high-contrast background for visualizing the cornea and aiding in the lamellar dissection of the cornea. The entire unit is sterile and disposable for convenience. The chamber is designed with a peripheral angle so that the surgeon can still use a regular set of lamellar dissection instruments with the disposable chamber. The design of the chamber allows the surgeon to firmly hold a 14–18 mm donor cornea on a bed of viscoelastic material, pressurize it, and cut it from the epithelial side. At the authors' eye center, they have built a metal holder to secure the whole AAC and increase its stability to work with the femtosecond laser system.

The authors have now explained the basic steps previously described[5] to prepare the corneoscleral disk onto the chamber:

First, disassemble the components of the Barron AAC and prepare the instruments on the table (Fig. 7.13). Prepare 2 syringes and fill them with desired fluid or air medium (i.e. Optisol GS solution and BSS). Connect the syringes to the 2 ports attached to the base of the AAC. Keep the pinch locks in the open position. Purge the first port with BSS and snap the pinch lock shut. Using Optisol GS solution, fill the second port until the fluid covers the base of the chamber. Leave the pinch lock in the open position. Apply viscoelastic material to the endothelial side of corneoscleral button. Place the corneoscleral button (Fig. 7.14) on the base of the AAC avoiding any air pockets under the graft once the corneoscleral button is mounted. Place the tissue retainer over the corneoscleral button (Fig. 7.15), aligning the guideposts; then, advance the tissue retainer to the bottom of the chamber base. Place the locking ring over the tissue retainer. While holding the tissue retainer with one hand, use the other hand to rotate the locking ring into the closed position (Fig. 7.16). The donor corneoscleral button is now securely in place. Infuse the Optisol GS solution through the irrigation port and shut the pinch lock once the desired pressure is achieved.

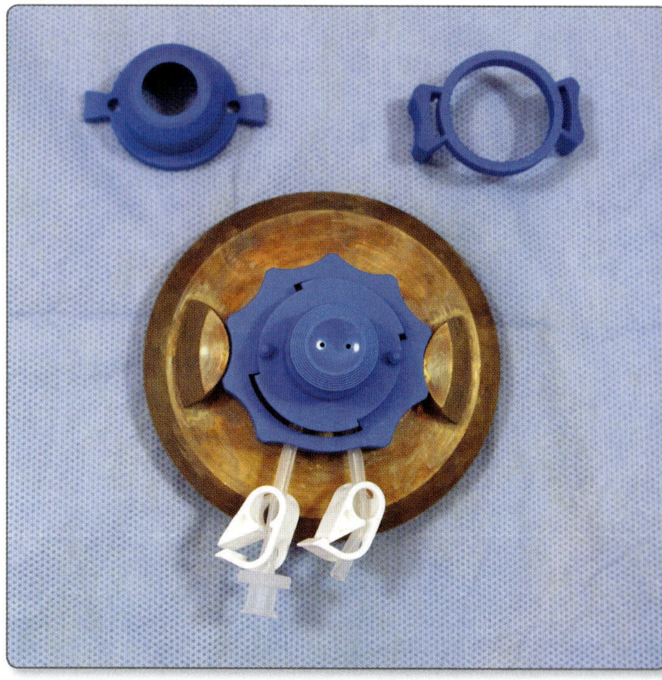

Fig. 7.13: Barron´s artificial anterior chamber disassembled with its three parts: the base, the locking ring and the tissue retainer

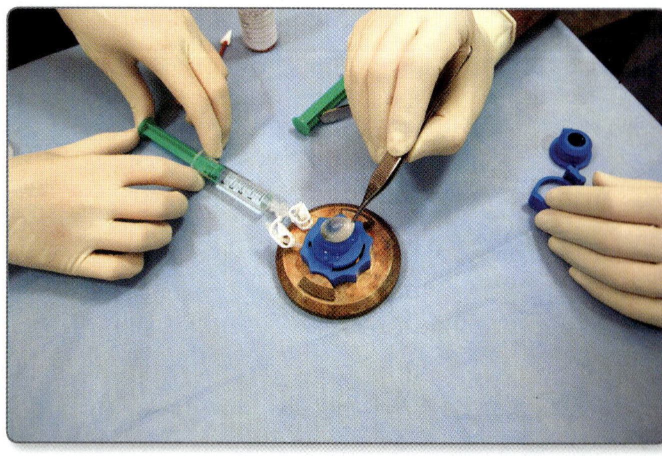

Fig. 7.14: Positioning of the tissue on the chamber base. Irrigating through one port while the other is pinched to avoid air bubbles inside the artificial anterior chamber

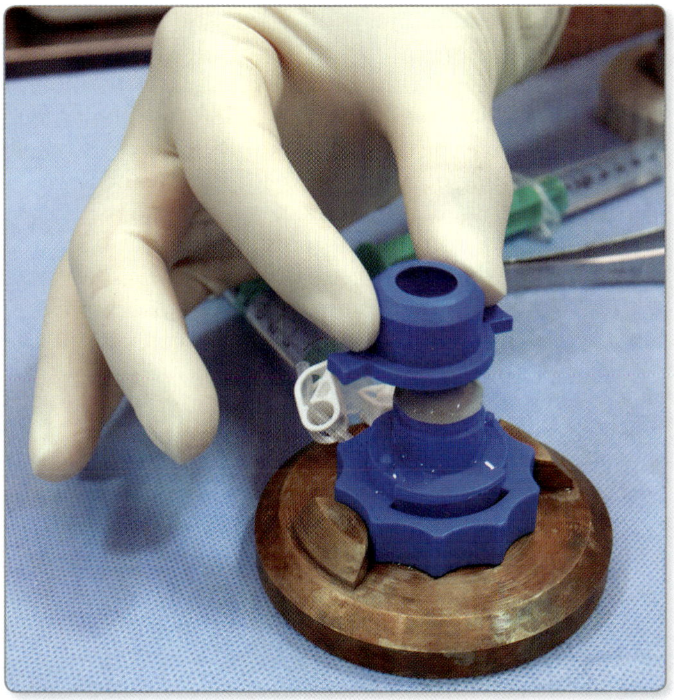

Fig. 7.15: Placing the locking ring when the tissue is properly centered. Do not touch the peripheral scleral rim to avoid decentering

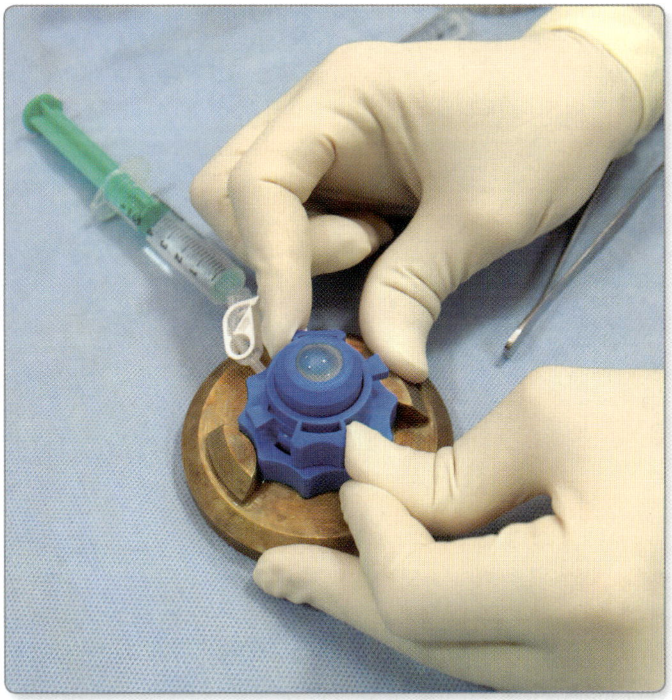

Fig. 7.16: Rotating firmly with both hands the locking ring to seal the artificial anterior chamber

Several modifications of this standard technique have been proposed and, recently, the use of dispersive viscoelastic agents[6] has given more stable results.

Like the other two disposable AAC, the Barron model is very simple to assemble and fits to all femtosecond laser system available.

HOW TO USE AN ARTIFICIAL ANTERIOR CHAMBER IN FEMSTOSECOND LASER-ASSISTED KERATOPLASTY

As authors have stated previously, a perfect contact between the donor surface and the femtosecond laser cone is critical to achieve a correct corneal tissue cutting profile. Authors have described how to mount the tissue in the AAC; it is a basic step that the majority of corneal surgeons know well from other corneal procedures as mentioned previously. But once the tissue is in the AAC, it must be positioned under the femtosecond laser and make contact with the applanation cone to perform the laser tissue cut. The authors have described the basics of their routine technique to perform this step with a femtosecond laser system.

The authors presently use the IntraLase™ iEK 150 kHz Femtosecond laser system and the Barron disposable AAC to hold the donor cornea. This laser system has a flat applanating cone that must come in contact with a minimum area of the cornea with a minimum pressure. The laser cone is retracted upward passively when contacting with the cornea and a sensor measures the pressure the laser cone is applying to the cornea. With a downward movement controlled by the joystick, we lower the laser arm, which increases the pressure on the tissue, and achieving tissue applanation. The pressure-monitoring sensor informs the surgeon by a screen light indicator how much pressure we are applying to the tissue. When the indicator is green, pressure is optimum; when it is yellow, the pressure is high but laser beam working is allowed. When the indicator is red, the pressure is out of working range and damage can occur. This is especially important when performing the cut in the recipient´s eye.

The AAC holding the tissue must be placed under the laser cone on a floor-secured table or we can use the patient stretcher. It is very important that either the stretcher or the table is fixed to avoid any small movements that can affect the precision of the laser cut. Laser system can take up to 2 minutes to complete some cutting patterns and during this time, no movement or displacement of the AAC must be allowed. To improve our operating procedure, we use a round heavy metal piece (Fig. 7.17) that fits perfectly to the AAC base, allowing us to hold it firmly in place and work safely.

When the AAC is well-positioned under the laser system, we move the laser arm to create a contact applanation area between the cone and the tissue. It is important to have a

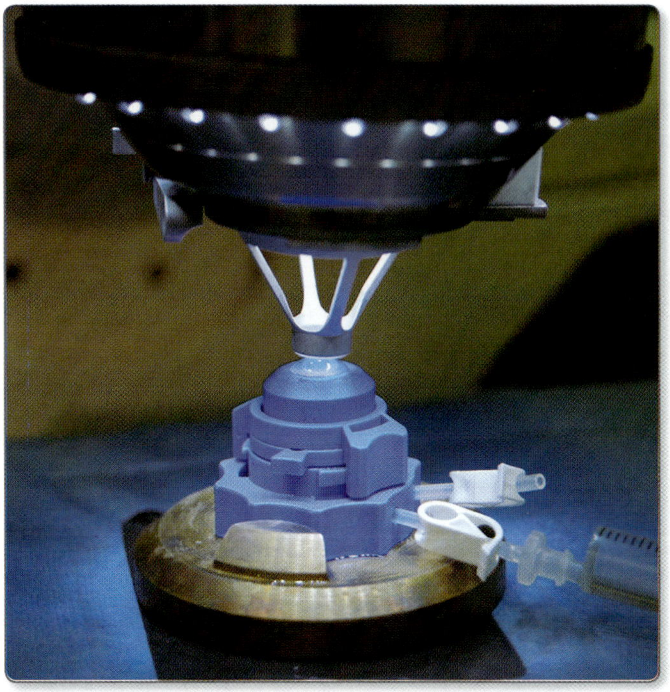

Fig. 7.17: Positioning of the artificial anterior chamber with the mounted tissue under the laser applanating cone

good aligning angle (Fig. 7.18) to avoid parallax errors that can create oval applanation areas. So we routinely check this angle between the cone and the tissue observing from a lateral position.

To achieve an optimum pressure inside the AAC, we can measure it previously with a tonometer, but we always check using the light indicators of the laser monitor. If pressure is too low, we inject more BSS using the syringe connected to one of the ports until the display is green; then we clamp the port. If pressure is too high and the light indicator is red, we lift the cone and recommend decreasing the pressure by opening the port. We do not open the port with the applanating cone pushing against the tissue because a sudden loss of pressure and collapse in the AAC can damage the endothelium if it comes in contact with the AAC base.

Once a good applanating area and correct pressure are achieved, centering of the tissue is the next step (Fig. 7.19). Usually we mark the center with a surgical pen. The centering can initially be performed by laterally moving the joystick and fine adjustments can then be performed using the centering software of the laser system. The laser beam is then ready to be activated and start the programed cutting pattern (Fig. 7.20). During this step we have to avoid any movement or displacement of the laser arm or the AAC.

COMPLICATIONS

We can have some complications when using an AAC to prepare the tissue with the femtosecond laser. They can be related to improper positioning of the donor onto the AAC device or may occur during the laser-tissue interaction.

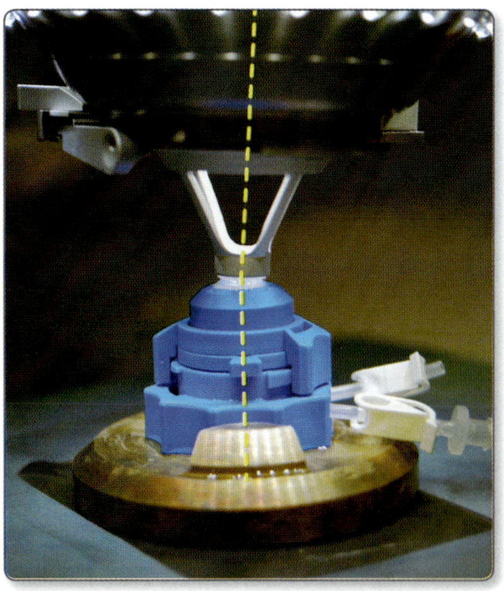

Fig. 7.18: Parallax angle between the laser axis and the artificial anterior chamber axis. It is important to have the minimum angle to achieve a perfect applanation area

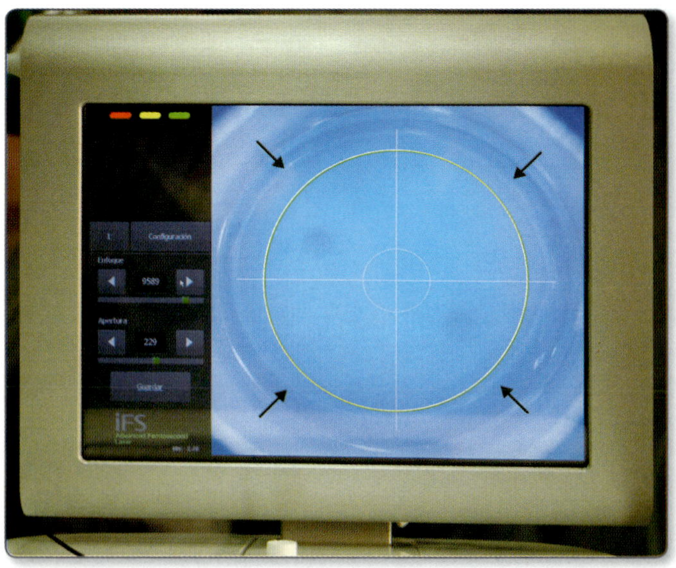

Fig. 7.19: Screen frame of the IntraLase™ iEK femtosecond laser system. We can see a yellow circle indicating the diameter of the cut in a standard vertical penetrating keratoplasty pattern, black arrows indicating the limits of the contact area, which must be out of the circular cutting pattern, and the three colored lights in the upper left corner that indicate the contact pressure level

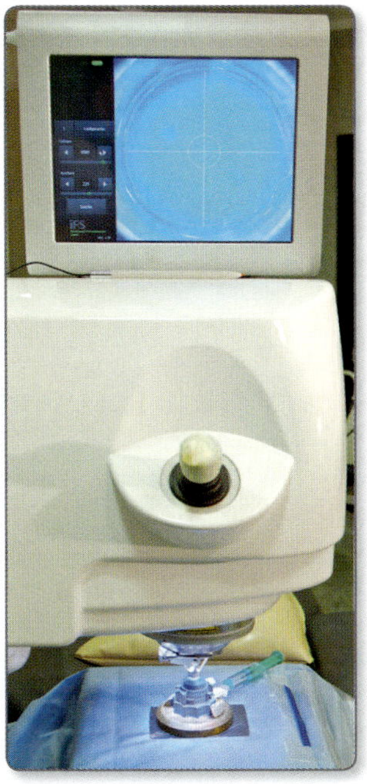

Fig. 7.20: Setup of the femtosecond laser when performing the cut of the cornea mounted in the artificial anterior chamber. A digital marking pen is available to make the appropriate changes in the centering touching the monitor screen. A sterile sheath covers the joystick to be safely manipulated by the surgeon

The main mistakes during positioning of the donor in the AAC are:

- Using a small diameter corneoscleral button: An adequate sealing of the chamber cannot be achieved or a sudden collapse can occur when applying the downward pressure with the laser cone.
- Decentering of the tissue: The desired diameter of the donor cutting cannot be obtained or peripheral cornea with *arcus senilis* or limbal area could be included in the cut.
- Collapsing of the chamber when manipulating the irrigation tubing or syringes: It can cause a contact between the endothelium and the plastic or metal base with subsequent damage to the endothelial monolayer, causing a primary graft failure or a lower-than-expected endothelial cell count for a penetrating posterior lamellar keratoplasty.

Other complications than can be observed during the step of femtosecond laser cut of the tissue are usually:

- Low pressure inside the AAC when the cone is applied: Careful increasing of the pressure must be performed. When the pressure is too low, laser treatment cannot be started, and if so, an irregular or oval cut can be obtained if a circular-vertical pattern has been programed or inaccurate in case of more advanced or complex patterns, such as zigzag, mushroom, top-hat or advanced combinations.
- High pressure inside the AAC: An insufficient contact with the laser cone and the tissue does not allow obtaining the desired cutting diameter. A different cutting angle between the donor and recipient can be obtained if there is a high disparity in pressure when performing the cut with non-applanating lasers.[7] The AAC must be checked and pressure gently adjusted.
- Decentering of the cutting pattern: Careful marking of the center of the cornea must be done previously and checking through the monitor screen or microscope must be performed prior to activating the laser beam.

CLINICAL PEARLS IN USING AN ARTIFICIAL ANTERIOR CHAMBER FOR FEMTO-KERATOPLASTY

- Ensure that the donor corneoscleral button has a wide rim. The diameter should be a minimum of 14–18 mm to guarantee a good seal around the AAC before the surgeon begins the tissue cutting. The surgeon should request this from the eye bank that prepares the donor buttons.
- Follow carefully all the steps when placing the tissue in the AAC avoiding any collapse.
- Check for adequate pressure inside the AAC.
- Make sure that the AAC is well positioned and fixed under the laser system.
- Use appropriate maneuvers to ensure proper centering of the cutting pattern in the corneal tissue.

REFERENCES

1. Meltendorf C, Schroeter J, Bug R, et al. Corneal trephination with the femtosecond laser. Cornea. 2006;25:1090-2.
2. Behrens A, Ellis K, Li L, et al. Endothelial lamellar keratoplasty using an artificial anterior chamber and a microkeratome. Arch Ophthalmol. 2003;121:503-8.
3. Wiley LA, Joseph MA, Springs CL. Tectonic lamellar keratoplasty utilizing a microkeratome and an artificial anterior chamber system. Cornea. 2002;21:661-3.
4. Robert PY, Adenis JP, Denis F, et al. Transmission of viruses through corneal transplantation. Clin Lab. 2005;51:419-23.
5. Rocha G, Bowler T. Use of a disposable artificial anterior chamber for trans-epithelial trephination and endothelial keratoplasty. Techniq Ophthalmol. 2007;5:21-6.
6. Iovieno A, Chowdhury V, Stevens JD, et al. Moorfields technique of donor cornea mounting for femtosecond-assisted keratoplasty: use of viscoelastic in the artificial anterior chamber. Ophthalmic Surg Lasers Imaging. 2012;43:348-50.
7. Sauer R, Seitz B, Mardin C, et al. Impact of intracameral pressure on donor cut angles in nonmechanical Er:YAG laser trephination for penetrating keratoplasty. Klin Monbl Augenheilkd. 2003;220:396-403.

Chapter

8

Femtosecond Laser-Assisted Penetrating Keratoplasty with IntraLase Technology (Use of the Different Technologies, Surgical Practical Pearls, Outcomes)

Jorge L Alió, Felipe Soria, Alfredo Vega, Ahmed A Abdou

CHAPTER OUTLINE

- Preoperative considerations when deciding
  - Indications
  - Preoperative evaluation
  - General considerations
  - Anesthesia
  - Ophthalmological examination
- Surgical procedure for corneal receptor
- Surgical procedure for corneal donor using the Moria artificial anterior chamber
- Overview of outcomes reported with the use of femtosecond-assisted penetrating keratoplasty
- Example of clinical cases

INTRODUCTION

By definition penetrating keratoplasty (PKP) refers to a corneal transplant, or graft, in which the entire thickness of the cornea is replaced.

The goal of every surgery is to restore the anatomy, functionality and cosmetic of the tissue. This goal is even more difficult when we are facing a corneal transplant where donor and recipient must be linked together like a puzzle and last for the lifetime of the patient.

Three mainstays are important in corneal transplant:

1. Election of the procedure: Penetrating keratoplasty or lamellar procedure.
2. Incision configuration.
3. Incision creation with femtosecond laser enabled keratoplasty.

In 1905, Eduard Zirm did the first full-thickness PKP near Prague.[1] Since then, the evolution in keratoplasty has been a slow process in comparison to other ophthalmic surgical techniques. By the mid of 1950, the introduction of steroids was one of the most important factors for success in this technique. Other advances like the introduction of nylon monofilament suture, ophthalmic viscosurgical devices, contact lenses, techniques for tissue preservation and tissue matching has contributed to an improvement of these procedures.

Other important advance has been the development of different surgical techniques. In 1921, Carrell and Eberling proposed a straight graft configuration, meanwhile in 1950; Barraquer described a series of patterns in which among that was the top-hat pattern.

In the 1970s, there was an increased interest in lamellar corneal transplantation[2] and in the last 10 years, corneal transplant surgery has been revolutionized with the development and refinement of lamellar transplants as well as with the introduction of femtosecond technology to this procedure.

Penetrating Keratoplasty versus Lamellar Procedures

The major criterion for the election of the technique is the consideration of the pathological portion of the cornea and the technical possibility in achieving the procedure election.

The technical description of lamellar techniques (anterior, deep lamellar or posterior) achieves to transplant only the pathological portion of the cornea.

The major benefits this entails are—the absence of potential corneal endothelial cell immune rejection, the conservation of corneal endothelial cell count, extraocular procedure and topical corticosteroids can usually be discontinued earlier, superior resistance to rupture of the globe after blunt trauma and sutures can be removed earlier.[1] Despite all of this, PKP is still one of the most chosen procedures when making a corneal transplant. The main advantages of PKP are—treatment of corneal conditions that involve the endothelium, penetrating corneal traumas and scars comprising the Descemet's membrane and a more familiar operative procedure for most surgeons.

Incision Configuration

As was discussed above, since the first PKP was done in 1905, the quest for the best incision type started. The main objectives of an incision in any corneal transplant is to achieve an excellent wound apposition between donor and recipient, to maintain the wound integrity with minimal suture tension (capacity of an equal 360° wound healing), preserve biomechanically the corneal structure and induce the minimal astigmatism possible.[3-5]

Several incisional patterns have been described from a straight to a zig-zag configuration. For the purpose of this chapter, we will name only the most common and which have submitted a better efficiency. In 1950, Barraquer recognized the advantages of a stepped incision[6] and also Busin published its results in 2003 demonstrating the optimization of postkeratoplasty refractive error with a substantially faster visual recovery with a wound construction based on the nut-and-bolt concept.[1,7]

Following these stepped incisional configuration is that different studies have shown that zig-zag and top-hat configurations are the most optimal.[3,4,8] In our experience, we share these findings and are our elections in PKP and deep anterior lamellar keratoplasty (DALKP) procedures.

Incision Creation with Femtosecond Laser Enabled Keratoplasty

In the era of femtosecond lasers, moreover, no matter which type of transplant technique the patients require (penetrating or lamellar), using the femtosecond laser enables a precise cut without damaging surrounding tissue. Femtosecond lasers exceed in accuracy, reproducibility and standardization, all very important objectives in order to achieve a perfect coupling.

Particularly, our experienced is based in the use of IntraLase 60 kHz that allows the possibility of the selection of three types of cutting patterns (Mushroom, Top-Hat and Zig-Zag) with the precise coupling between donor and recipient. The precise coupling pattern brings the obvious benefit of a tighter seal in conjunction with sutures. Another possible benefits in the use of femtosecond laser technology is the photodisruption of corneal tissue may stimulate more rapid and stronger the healing of the incision.[9]

FEMTOSECOND LASER-ASSISTED PENETRATING KERATOPLASTY

Preoperative Considerations

Indications[1,10]

- Corneal edema associated to corneal scarring or with a very long and chronic evolution.
- *Deep stromal scars caused by*: Trauma, severe infectious process of any etiology and hydrops in keratoconus. In the case of hydrops, the rupture of Descemet's membrane makes impossible to find the plane of cleavage in order to perform a lamellar technique.
- Immunological disorders associated with corneal perforation (rheumatoid arthritis and Mooren's ulcer).
- Active infective process (any etiology). The only limitation is the possibility of the femtosecond laser to overstep dense opacities and blood vessels.
- Recurrent transplant rejection.

In case of corneal perforation less than 3 mm and if the corneal thickness is acceptable, the procedure can be done in which case the perpendicular docking closes the perforation during the femtosecond dissection (Fig. 8.1).

Preoperative Studies

As the main objective of this procedure is to reestablish the best visual acuity possible, the clinician must perform a complete ophthalmological evaluation having the absolute certainty of the potential vision of the patient. On the other hand, the clinician must explain to the patient about the expectations in terms of the visual acuity that the patient will achieve after the surgery and also to take into consideration the possible complications and the fact of a prolonged postoperative treatment. The patients must know that they will reach their complete visual potential

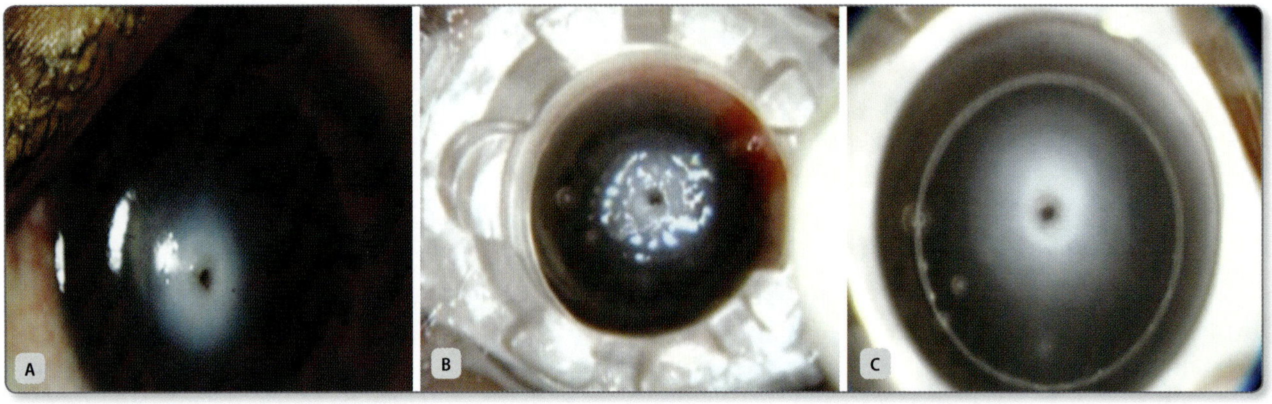

Fig. 8.1: The method to achieve a perfect docking in a perforated recipient eye. First the anterior chamber was filled with cohesive ophthalmic viscosurgical device (OVD) and then the femtosecond procedure was done without any complication

after the sutures are removed and a refractive treatment is instituted and this usually will take at least 9 months, in this way, the patient will not have false expectations or be frustrated by the visual acuity achieved in the immediate postoperative period.

General Considerations

The preoperative assessment should always include the consultation of general medicine or anesthesiologist department. Those patients with high risk of corneal graft rejection, in which an immune suppression therapy will be institute after the procedure, should also have a blood test analysis including serology, renal and liver function. Specific exploration about bleeding disorders and related drugs must be recognized. Patients receiving anticoagulants are advised to cease 7 days before the surgery the intake of their medication because of the increased risk of expulsive hemorrhage.

Anesthesia

During the clinical evaluation of the patient we can have an insight of the type of anesthesia that the patient will need. It is essential to take in the consideration the systemic condition of the patient and age with the aim of providing patient comfort, safety of the procedure and low rate of complications.

It is mandatory for children that general anesthesia should be used. In our experience, young and elderly patients may be properly handled by local anesthesia and moderate intravenous (IV) sedation.

Local anesthesia in a PKP case is either retrobulbar or peribulbar depending on the surgeon or anesthesiology preference or experience. Anesthesia should accomplish total oculomotor muscle akinesia and anesthesia orbicularis muscle total paralysis should be obtained by a facial nerve block. As PKP is an open sky globe procedure, thus, totally dependent of changes of intraocular pressures (IOPs), our main concern is to avoid an expulsive hemorrhage, thus we must consider the types of anesthesia to use.

As a routine in our practice, we perform the following approach:

Local anesthesia (peribulbar): Peribulbar anesthesia is the gold standard for our keratoplasty procedures. In our experience, the combination of lidocaine and bupivacaine 50/50 in 5 mL is sufficient to achieve both akinesia and anesthesia. There is some controversy on when to perform the anesthesia, while some authors consider the peribulbar anesthesia after the femtosecond procedure,[10] in our experience is better to do it before, to avoid having to increase the volume inside the orbit or mobilizing the patient to another operating theater in case that the eye is inadvertently perforated during the femtosecond procedure.

Regional anesthesia (facial nerve block): Additionally, we also performed as routine a block in the facial nerve so that the akinesia of the orbicularis muscle does not exert added pressure over the speculum increasing in this way the IOP. This anesthesia also contributes to the anesthetic effect provided by the peribulbar anesthesia thus helping to decrease the volume of the latest into the orbit.

General anesthesia: As in every ophthalmology surgery, every child must undergo surgery under general anesthesia. Adolescents and elderly patients may be considered for this type of anesthesia also. We suggest the following conditions:

- Extreme patient anxiety
- Inability of the patient to cooperate with the surgical team
- Inability to provide satisfactory local or topical anesthesia
- Known allergy to local or topical anesthetic medications
- The presence of disorders that may be better managed under general anesthesia, i.e. severe back pain, postural problems, etc.

Sedation: Routine sedation in every case is used, where obviously general anesthesia is not the indication.

The technical aspects of each type of anesthetic procedure are not covered because it is beyond the subject matter of the present chapter.

Ophthalmological Examination

- *Topography*: Although is not mandatory study for the surgery, it is, for the diagnosis of the pathology and relevant examination for the history clinic.
- *Pachymetry*:
  - *Anterior optical coherence tomography (OCT)*: It is a mandatory preoperative study. Measuring the central and peripheral corneal thickness will allow us to determine the parameters of the incisions for our surgical planning. It is also important to note the OCT capacity to obtain the dimensions (depth and longitude) of the opacities and evaluate the possibility of femtosecond to breakthrough them (Figs 8.2 and 8.3).
  - *Ultrasonic pachymetry*: The day of the surgery, before the femtosecond laser procedure, measurements with this technology should be conducted. Normally, the pathological corneas to be transplanted including certain changes in the thickness, so that this method provides us a double check measurement. The sequence for taking the measurements is suggested as following: Starting in the center and placing the probe in the intended zone of the incisions, approximately in the mid-periphery (between 7 and 9 mm) of the cardinal points following the mid-periphery obliquely to the cardinal points, in total, we suggest at least 9 measurements. This data should be compared with the OCT pachymetry. In our experience, we suggest not to perform the femtosecond for the dissection of the cornea when the thickness is below 350 microns because of overlapping of the incisions.

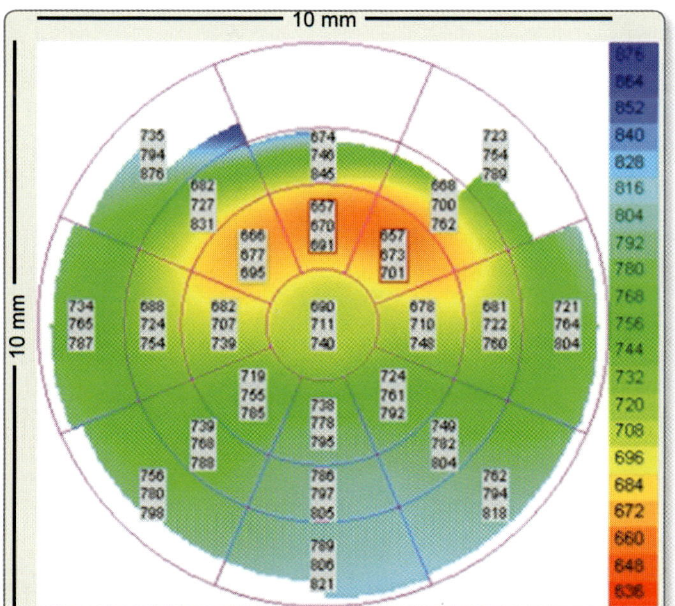

Range (mm)	Minimum	Average	Maximum
0 – 2	690	711	740
2–5	657	716	795
5–7	668	746	845
7–10	721	782	876

Fig 8.2: The pachymetry map of a patient with bullous keratopathy that will undergo femtosecond penetrating keratoplasty procedure

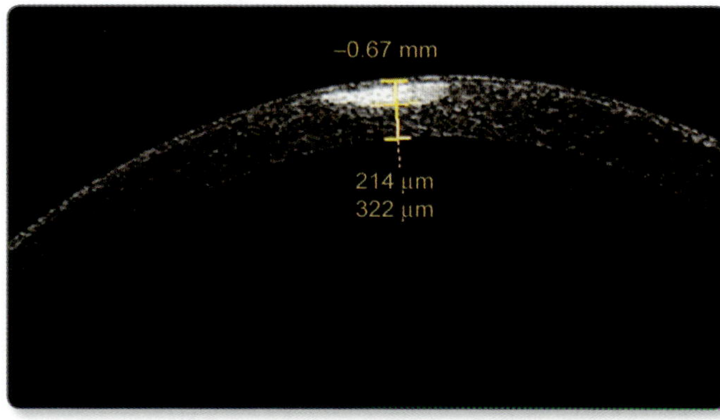

Fig. 8.3: Anterior segment OCT of a patient with anterior corneal scar with history of a previous infectious keratitis

SURGICAL PROCEDURE FOR CORNEAL RECEPTOR

Femtosecond technology allow us to perform different staggered patterns that otherwise cannot be achieved with a standard corneal trephine. These designs will result in an excellent apposition of the tissue, which will lead to a rapid wound healing and an earlier removal of the suture with a faster recovery of the patients. IntraLase technology allows 3 different types of corneal pattern incisions. Each types of incision are described below giving the following details: Indications, benefits, disadvantages and settings of the laser machine.

Pattern Shape Selection (Figs 8.4A to C)

Zig-Zag Pattern

Indications:

- *Any case*:
  - *Benefits*: Having the experience in corneal three plane incisions during cataract surgery is that our

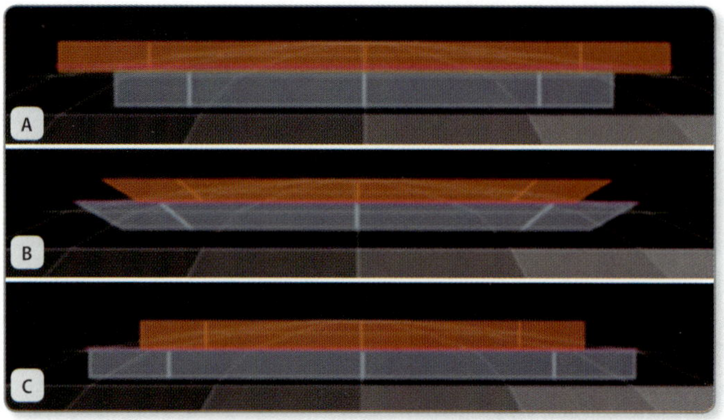

Figs 8.4A to C: Dissection patterns: (A) Zig-zag (B) Top-hat (C) Mushroom

preference for a PKP is choosing the zig-zag pattern. This kind of shape simulates two grooves that in the correct angle allow the maximum opposition for leakage. As an added value, the maximum apposition established allows an untight suture pattern with the refractive benefits that this gives.

- *Disadvantages*: Not possible to use this pattern if peripheral thickening exists.
- *IntraLase settings sample*:

Ring lamellar cut:	On
Depth in cornea:	300
Outer diameter:	9.0
Inner diameter:	7.6
Energy:	1.80
Tangential spot separation:	4
Radial spot separation:	4
Full lamellar cut:	Off
Anterior side cut:	On
Posterior depth:	320
Anterior diameter:	8.2
Energy:	2.10
Cut position 1:	0
Cut angle 1:	360
Cut position 2:	180
Cut angle 2:	0
Anterior side cut angle:	45
Anterior side cut spot separation:	3
Anterior side cut layer separation:	2
Depth in glass:	50
Posterior side cut:	On
Anterior depth:	280
Posterior diameter:	8.9
Posterior energy:	2.10
Posterior post depth:	

i. Thinnest pachymetry point: 125 μ
ii. 70% of the thinnest pachymetry point
iii. Cornea edema: 50% of the thinnest pachymetry point

Posterior side cut angle:	45
Posterior side cut spot separation:	3
Posterior side cut layer separation:	2
Alignment incisions:	Off

Barrel incision type described by Dr Neuhann (Fig. 8.4B) has the same characteristics and indications as zig-zag pattern, but in our practice we do not use it because of the good results presented with the latter.

Top-Hat Pattern

- *Indications*:
  - Central scars
  - Posterior peripheral scars
  - Corneal edema
  - Peripheral superior corneal thickening more than 350 μ.
- *Benefits*: Larger amounts of corneal stroma and endothelium graft will be transplanted.
- *Disadvantages*: The straight-edge-to-straight-edge configuration is associated with delayed, weak and incomplete healing of the donor-host junction.
- *IntraLase settings sample*:

Ring lamellar cut:	On
Depth in cornea:	280
Outer diameter:	9.3
Inner diameter:	8.3
Energy:	1.80
Tangential spot separation:	4
Radial spot separation	4
Spiral start:	Out
Full lamellar cut:	Off
Anterior side cut:	On
Posterior depth:	300
Anterior diameter:	8.4
Energy:	2.10
Cut position 1:	0
Cut angle 1:	360
Cut position 2:	180
Cut angle 2:	0
Anterior side cut angle:	90
Anterior side cut spot separation:	3
Anterior side cut layer separation:	2
Depth in glass:	50
Posterior side cut:	On
Anterior depth:	260
Posterior diameter:	9.2
Posterior energy:	2.10
Posterior post depth:	

i. Thinnest pachymetry point: 125 μ
ii. 70% of the thinnest pachymetry point
iii. Cornea edema: 50% of the thinnest pachymetry point

Posterior side cut angle	90
Posterior side cut spot separation	3
Posterior side cut layer separation:	2
Alignment incisions:	Off

Mushroom Pattern

- *Indications*:
  - Central scars
  - Superficial peripheral scars
  - Keratoconus
  - Peripheral inferior corneal thickening more than 350 μ
- *Benefits*: Larger amounts of corneal tissue is added to the thin periphery and minimizes the extraction of healthy endothelium.
- *Disadvantages*: The straight-edge-to-straight-edge configuration is associated with delayed, weak and incomplete healing of the donor-host junction.
- *IntraLase settings sample*:

Ring lamellar cut:	On
Depth in cornea:	280
Outer diameter:	8.5
Inner diameter:	7.5
Energy:	1.90
Tangential spot separation:	4
Radial spot separation:	4
Spiral start:	Out
Full lamellar cut:	Off
Anterior side cut:	On
Posterior depth:	300
Anterior diameter:	8.4
Energy:	2.05
Cut position 1:	0
Cut angle 1:	360
Cut position 2:	180
Cut angle 2:	0
Anterior side cut angle:	90
Anterior side cut spot separation:	3
Anterior side cut layer separation:	2
Depth in glass:	50
Posterior side cut:	On
Anterior depth:	260
Posterior diameter:	7.6
Posterior energy:	2.05

Posterior post depth:

i. Thinnest pachymetry point: 125 μ
ii. 70% of the thinnest pachymetry point
iii. Cornea edema: 50% of the thinnest pachymetry point

Posterior side cut angle	90
Posterior side cut spot separation:	3
Posterior side cut layer separation:	2
Alignment incisions:	Off

When all the settings are rationally established in the IntraLase by the surgeon and the patient is lying in the couch, our routine approach is the following:

- Select the optical wheel of the IntraLase to position D and focus on the receptor cornea (Fig. 8.5).
- Verify with a caliper the white to white measurement (Figs 8.6A and B). This will allow assessing if the diameter that was programed in the femtosecond parameters is in concordance with the diameter of the cornea.
- *Ultrasonic pachymetry measurements*: Starting in the center and placing the probe in the intended zone of the incisions, approximately in the mid-periphery of the cardinal points following the mid-periphery oblicually to the cardinal points (between 7 mm and 9 mm), in total, we suggest at least nine measurements. This data should be compared with the OCT pachymetry. In case that corneal edema is confirmed, we have to remember to calculate the posterior depth of the posterior side cut to 50% as mentioned above (Figs 8.7A and B).
- With a marker, proceed to check the center of the cornea for an accurate centration of the dissection with the femtosecond (Figs 8.8A to C).
- *Eye fixation with corneal suction ring*: The easiest way to achieve a good suction of the eye ball is to have the assistant hold the inferior eye lid, and the surgeon will hold the upper lid, the inferior border of the ring will gently but firmly placed over the inferior globe, after this, the ring will be placed over the sclera, making sure to achieve the best symmetrical position. As soon the best position is achieved suction will be demanded (Fig. 8.9).
- *Cone positioning and perpendicular docking*: One of the most important steps in this procedure is to achieve a perfect docking. When lowering down the cone the optical wheel will be changed to position 2 (Fig. 8.10) and

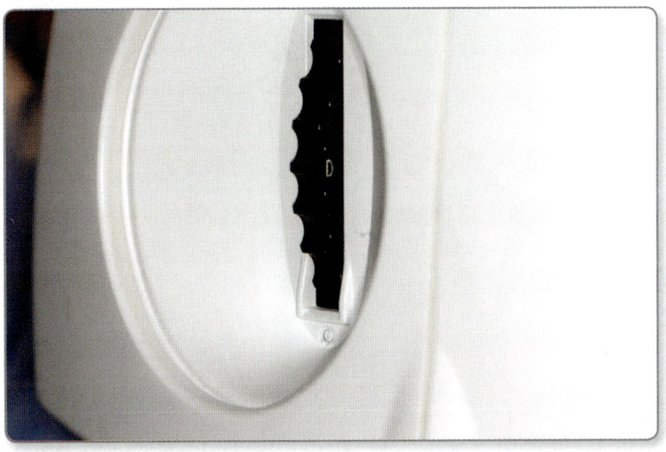

Fig. 8.5: Optical wheel of the IntraLase to position D and focus on the receptor cornea

the key orientation will be the circular light pattern of the illumination mechanism projected over the cornea. We suggest to always call these step perpendicular docking, because we emphasize in the surgeons mind the correct positioning of the cone over the cornea. When contact is made with the cornea, a meniscus will be seen starting from the center and moving to the periphery in an equal way. If the meniscus is not even, gently corrections can be made to the side moving the suction ring where the meniscus is greater, but NEVER the joystick in the X/Y direction. When the meniscus left behind the cutting pattern, the clip can be opened (Figs 8.11A to D).

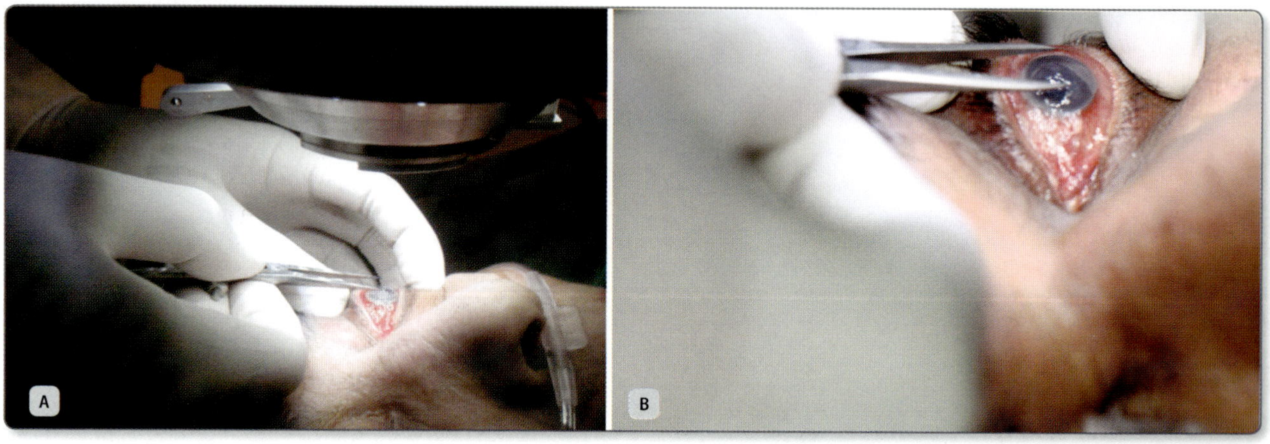

Figs 8.6A and B: The measurement of the white-to-white distance in order to plan the diameter of the dissection with the IntraLase

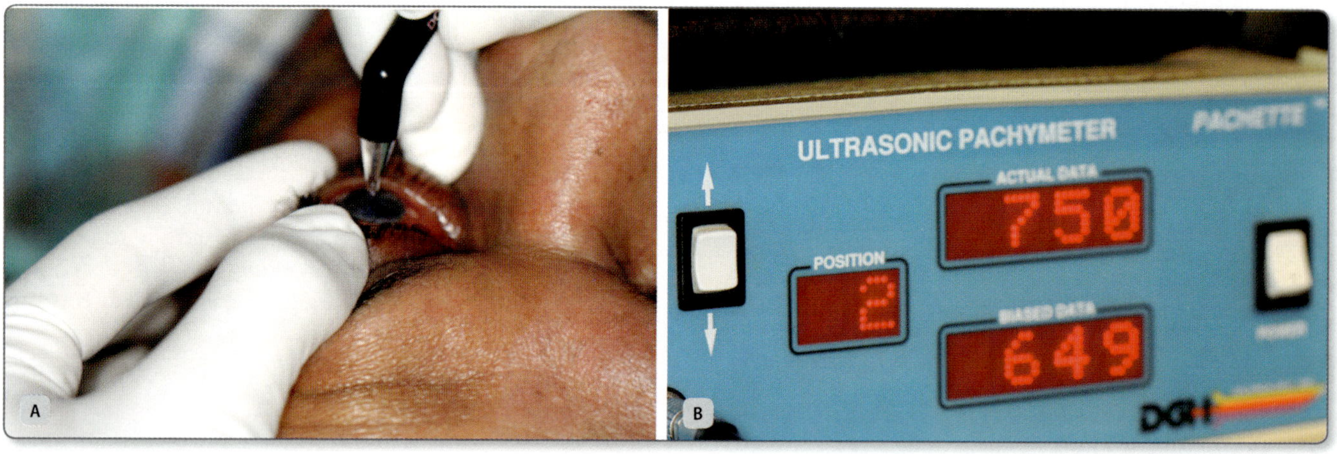

Figs 8.7A and B: (A) Pachymetric measurements; (B) Lecture of pachymetry measurement

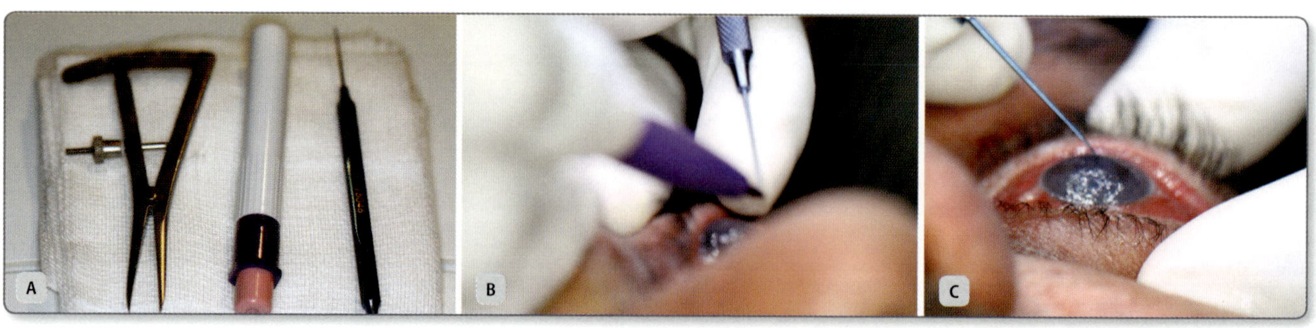

Figs 8.8A to C: Instruments for corneal marking is in (B and C) Showing how the center of the cornea is marked in order to assess a better centration of the femtosecond dissection

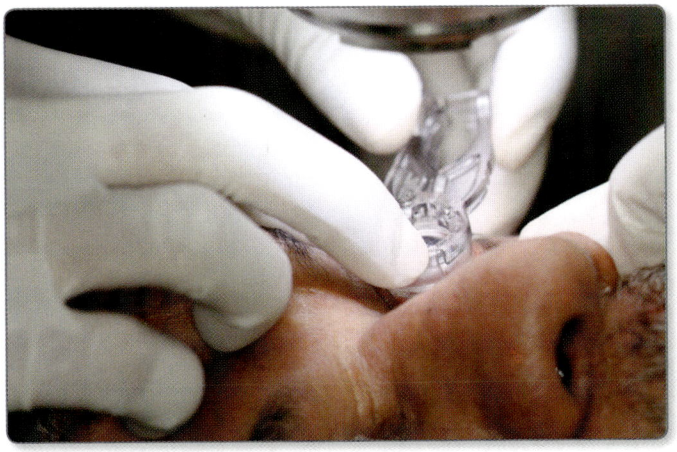

Fig. 8.9: The technique to achieve a good suction of the eye ball

Fig. 8.10: Position 2 for a correct visualization during docking process

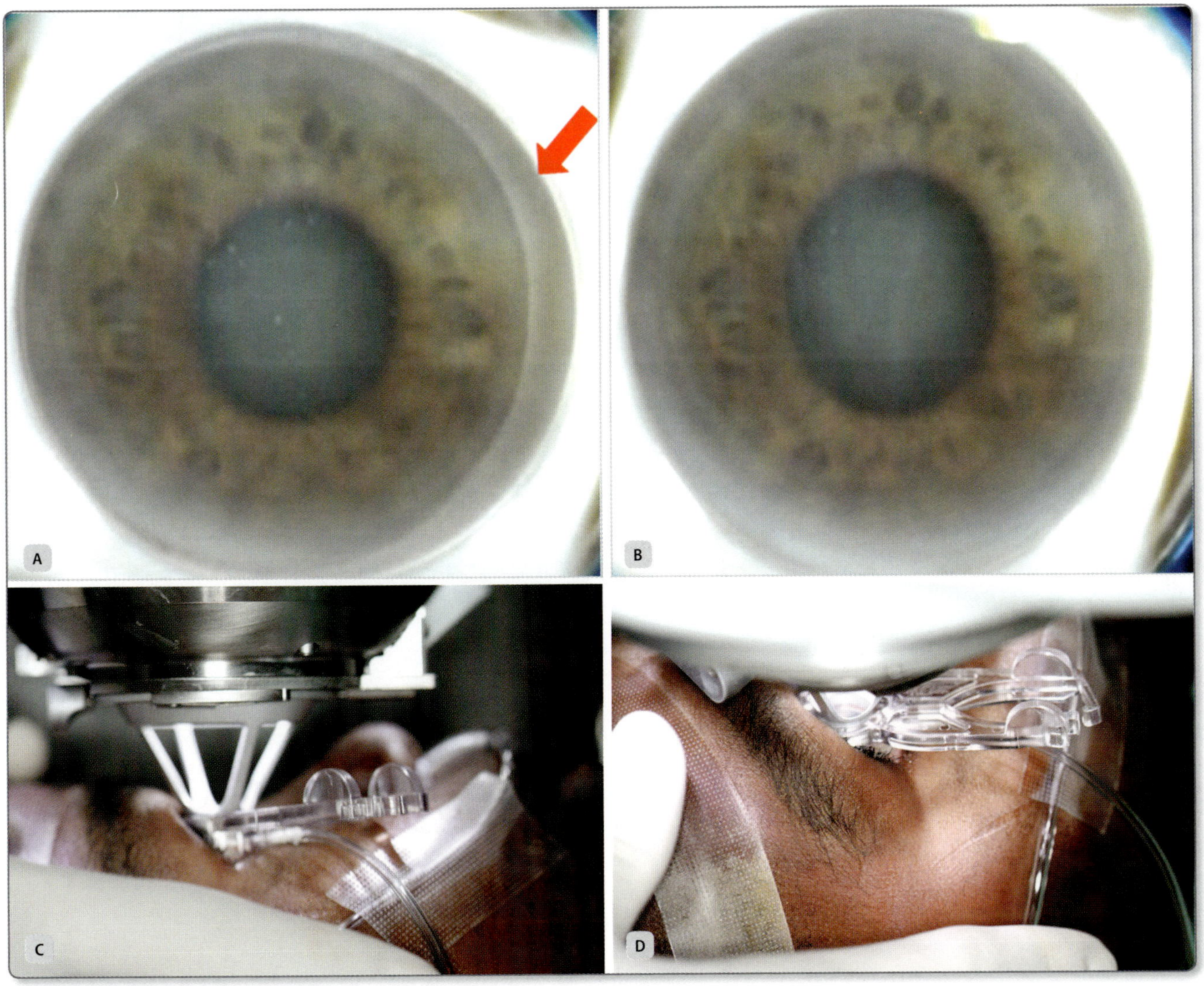

Figs 8.11A to D: (A) An uneven docking with the presence of meniscus in the right side of the image (Solid red arrow); (B) An adequate docking with complete absence of meniscus and the green light ON which means that the IntraLase system is ready to start with the dissection; (C) Perpendicular docking; (D) Clip opening when the meniscus is left behind on order to fix the laser-cone-suction ring-eye globe system

- *Centration of the dissection*: After the suction ring is fixated into the eye globe the assistant will center the dissection circle from the screen of the IntraLase on the mark that was previously done by the surgeon in the cornea (Fig. 8.12).
- *Pressing the foot pedal*: During this step, it is essential that all personnel in the operation room (OR) stand still making sure that no one touches the operating table or the IntraLase. Also assure that all cell phones are off.
  - *Normal view*: Depending on the patterns, the laser always starts the cuts from posterior to anterior, so what the surgeon must see is the presence of the bubbles generated by the laser in the deep stromal (Fig. 8.12).
  - *Abnormal view*: Bubbles in anterior chamber—if at the moment when the foot pedal is pressed, the surgeons notice the presence of bubbles in the anterior chamber, the procedure should be aborted and a new setting of the parameter changing the depth of the posterior side cut should be performed.
- The eye is patched and then the patient is transferred to a stretcher and taken to the OR where the procedure will be completed. In our settings this is easy, safe and fast because we have a door leading directly to the OR. Ideally, the surgical extraction of the cornea receptor starts meanwhile the donor cornea procedure has been done. Experience allows us to do both procedures parallel and when the surgeon requires the donor cornea these one will be ready.

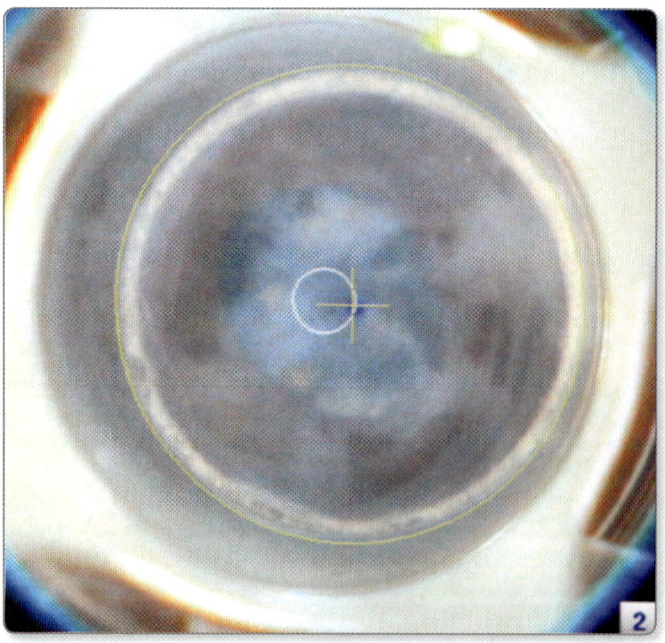

Fig. 8.12: Laser centration coinciding with corneal marking and incision creation

- Some key features that the surgeon should have taken into account are that separating the tissue previously dissected with the femtosecond can be achieved with a Sinskey's hook without needing a corneal trephine or knife. We suggest separating the corneas with the Sinskey's hook all 360° beginning in the upper side of the pattern and then continue with the deeper side. Once, this is performed the surgeon will continue with his/her habitual standard PKP procedure.

SURGICAL PROCEDURE FOR CORNEAL DONOR IN THE MORIA ARTIFICIAL ANTERIOR CHAMBER

During this procedure, the patient is kept in the OR where the recipient tissue is being removed. Ideally, perform this procedure before the surgeon begins with the surgery in the patient.

Setting up the Materials

Using aseptic technique, a table with wheels should be covered with a sterile field where the following instruments will be placed (Fig. 8.13):

- Donor corneal tissue (Fig. 8.14)
- Medicine cup with 10 mL of chlorhexidine
- Medical cup with 50 mL of balanced salt solution (BSS)
- Artificial anterior chamber (AAC)
- Forceps
- Caliper
- Surgical sponge
- Barraquer's tonometer
- 10 mL syringe.

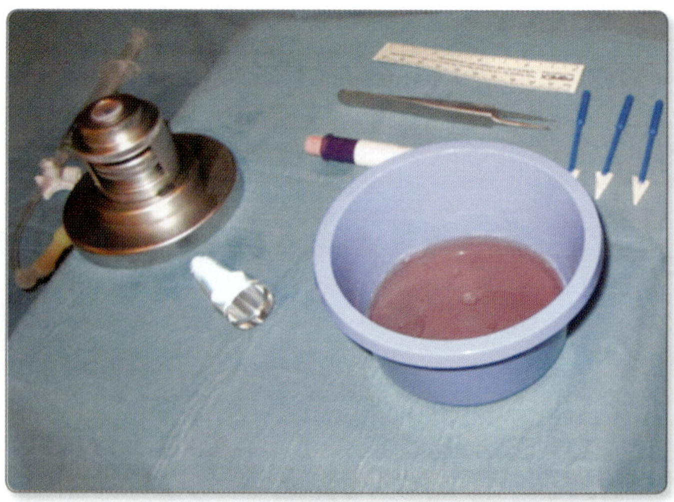

Fig. 8.13: The materials that are used as routine for the preparation of the corneal donor

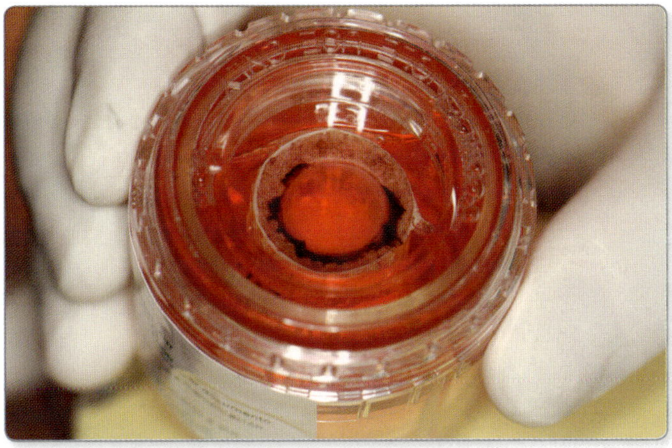

Fig. 8.14: Human corneal donor

Setting up the Sclerocorneal Donor in the Anterior Artificial Chamber and Proceeding with the IntraLaser Procedure

The procedure begins with a 5-minute surgical scrub technique followed by the placement of sterile gown and gloves.

- Connect the infusion IV line with the three way stopcock AAC.
- Fill-up the syringe with 10 mL of BSS and connect it to infusion IV line injecting BSS until the concave superior part of the piston is filled with BSS.
- Place sclerocorneal donor graft on the piston with the endothelium facing down using the forceps. Achieve a good centration making sure that no sclera is over the concave part of the piston (Fig. 8.15A).

Hold the graft with the forceps, and with the other hand, injects BSS in order to eliminate any air bubble. Gently, movements of the graft can be done to achieve the elimination of air bubbles. When this is achieved place the three-way stopcock in the position "closed" (Fig. 8.15B).

- Fit the anterior chamber cover over the graft and lock it in place with a 15° clockwise turn (Fig. 8.15C).
- Elevate the piston in order to tighten the chamber to the base and fixate the sclerocorneal rim (Fig. 8.15D).
- Measure the IOP with the Barraquer's tonometer to make sure that an adequate pressure is present in the sclerocorneal rim (Fig. 8.16).
- Place the table below the femtosecond and using the same cone that was used in the cornea of the patient, thus, the incisions must match precisely (Fig. 8.17).

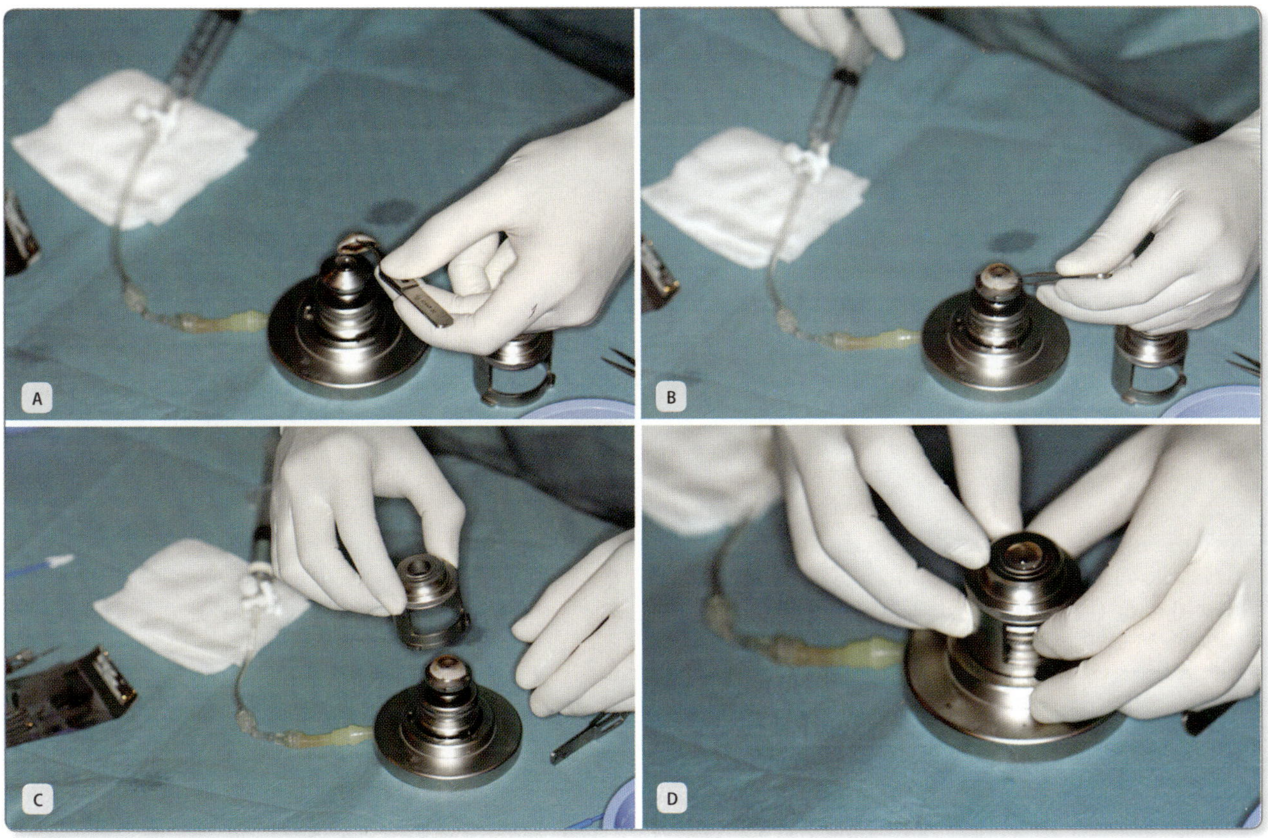

Figs 8.15A to D: Setting up the sclerocorneal donor in the anterior artifical chamber: (A) Placement of the sclerocorneal donor graft on the piston; (B) Injection of BSS with contralateral hand meanwhile positioning the graft on the piston and (C and D) Fitting of the anterior chamber

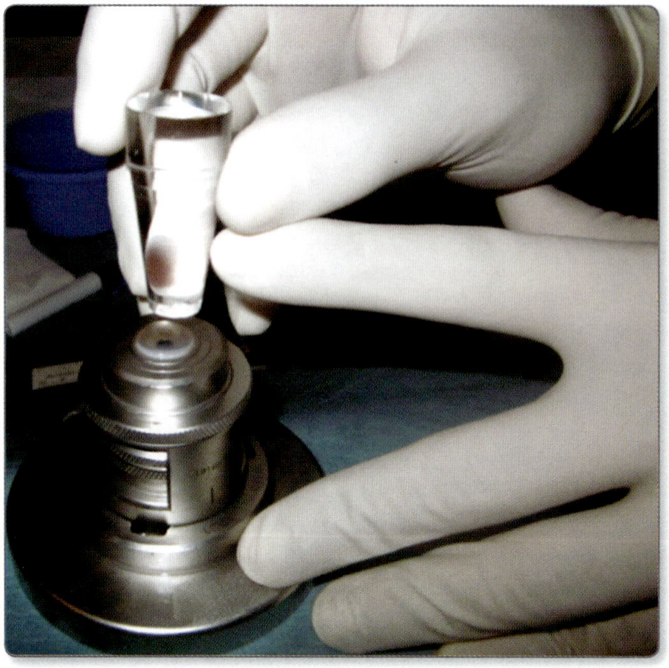

Fig. 8.16: The pressure inside the sclerocorneal rim is measured with the Barraquer´s tonometer

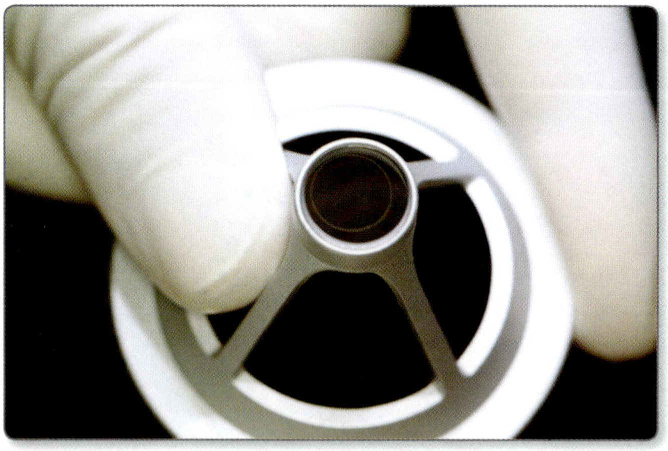

Fig. 8.17: The laser mark in the cone used early in the receptor. The same cone MUST be used in the corneal graft pattern

- Select the optical wheel of the IntraLase to position D and focus on the sclerocorneal rim.
- With a marker, proceed to mark the center of the cornea in order to achieve an adequate centration of the dissection.
- Make sure that the three-way stopcock is in position "closed".
- *Cone positioning and perpendicular docking (Fig. 8.18)*: When placing down the cone, the optical wheel of the IntraLase will be changed to position 2 and the key orientation will be the circular light pattern of the illumination mechanism projected over the cornea. We suggest to always call these step perpendicular docking, because we emphasize in the surgeons mind the correct positioning of the cone. When contact is made with the cornea, ask the assistant in the IntraLase to center the dissection on the mark that was previously done by the surgeon. Sometimes, if a small bubble was left inside the ACC, the procedure can also be centered in the bubble as usually it will be found in the center of the endothelium side of the sclerocorneal rim (Fig. 8.19). Finish the perpendicular docking until the meniscus is even or completely disappear. If the meniscus is not even, gently corrections can be made to the side where the meniscus is greater. When the meniscus is left behind and the green light is turned on, correct docking is achieved.

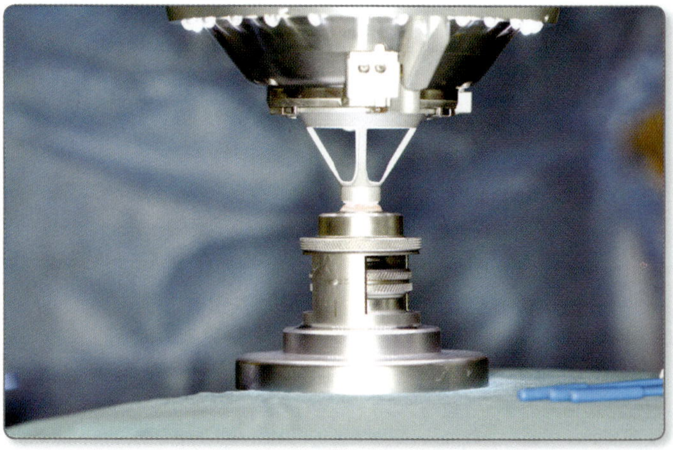

Fig. 8.18: Corneal graft docking

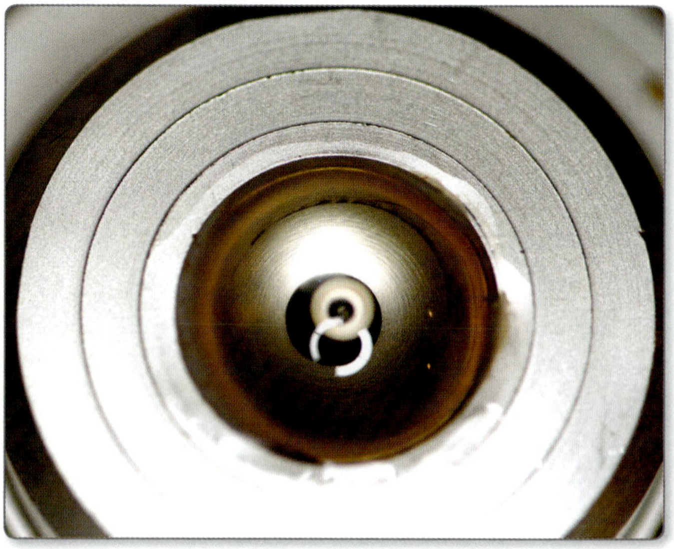

Fig. 8.19: An air bubble in the center of the endothelium that will not compromise an optimal cutting and helps as a reference of the corneal centration

- Double check together with the assistant that the correct pattern was designed (preview pattern in the IntraLase).
- Pressing the foot pedal:
  - *Normal view*: Depending on the patterns, the laser always starts the cuts from posterior to anterior, so what the surgeon must see in the first instance in the is the formation of air bubbles inside the AAC (Fig. 8.20).
  - *Abnormal view*: Uneven dissection pattern—the procedure should not be stopped but the surgeon must have in the consideration that the part of the cornea that was not properly dissected will not be easily removed from the sclera.
- *Undocking*: The elevation of the cone should be done slowly to observe the behavior of the donor cornea. If it's observed that the cornea is collapsing, BSS must be injected.
- Releasing the anterior chamber cover requires of very slow movements, the same as when lowering the piston. Doing both of these steps requires concomitantly the injection of BSS thus the corneal does not collapse. This avoids the creation of striae and probably loss of endothelial cells.
- The corneal graft is placed in the medical cap with chlorhexidine and it's taken to the OR for its implantation (Fig. 8.21).

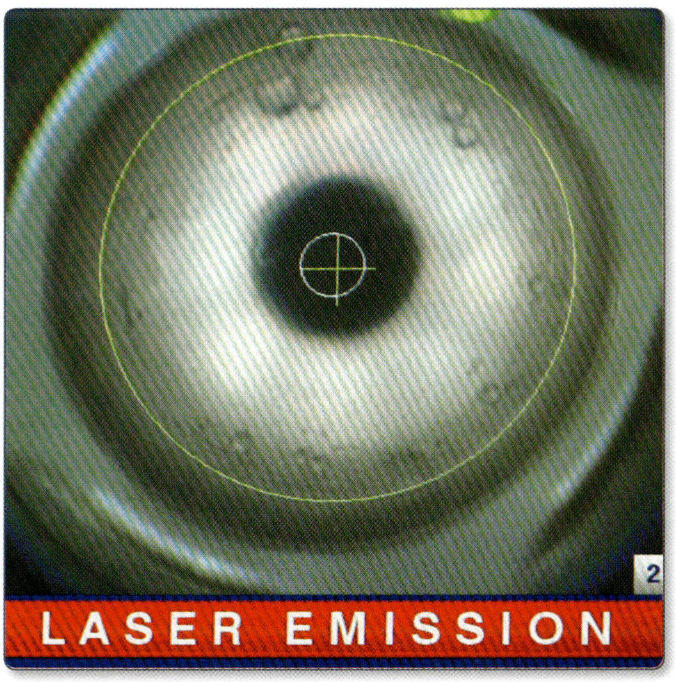

Fig. 8.20: Bubbles seeing in the artificial anterior chamber. In this step, the bubbles are demonstrating the optimal cut initiating from the posterior corneal graft

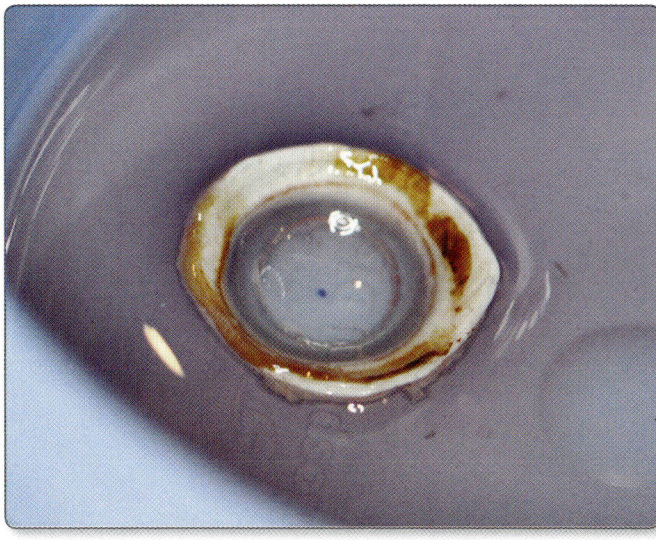

Fig. 8.21: The corneal donor graft with the central marking, with the cutting pattern in the chlorhexidine solution

- Once in the OR, the donor cornea can be dissected from the sclera rim by using an inverted Sinskey's hook. If an even dissection pattern was achieved with the femtosecond, grasping the sclera rim with a forceps and dissecting with the inverted Sinskey's hook around the 360° of the incision with the sclerocorneal rim over the donor cap, should be enough to get the corneal lenticule away from the sclera rim (Figs 8.22A to C). Afterward, the surgeon will continue with his habitual standard PKP procedure.

Outcomes

As for common indications for the conventional PKP like advanced Fuchs' dystrophy, severe pseudophakic bullous keratopathy, extensive trauma, corneal amyloidosis and severe keratoconus, the femtosecond laser assisted PKP (FSLAPKP) has been done with high efficacy and safety outcome[11,12] (Figs 8.23A and B). Not only the usual indications but FSLAPKP could be superior to PKP in case of repeated PKP and globe trauma with corneal laceration.[13,14]

Femtosecond laser-assisted penetrating keratoplasty (FSLAPKP) is highly safe and enables faster suture removal with better refractive and visual outcomes than the conventional PKP.[12,15] Farid et al.[16] published a comparative result between FSLAPKP (zig-zag pattern) and PKP concerning refractive and visual outcomes. Significant differences in the average postoperative astigmatism between the both groups after the first month *($P = 0.013$)* and the third one *($P = 0.018$)* were reported. By the third month, the average astigmatism was 3D in the zig-zag group and 4.46D in the conventional group. Significant differences in best spectacle-corrected visual acuity (BSCVA) were achieved after the first month *($P = 0.0003$)* and the third

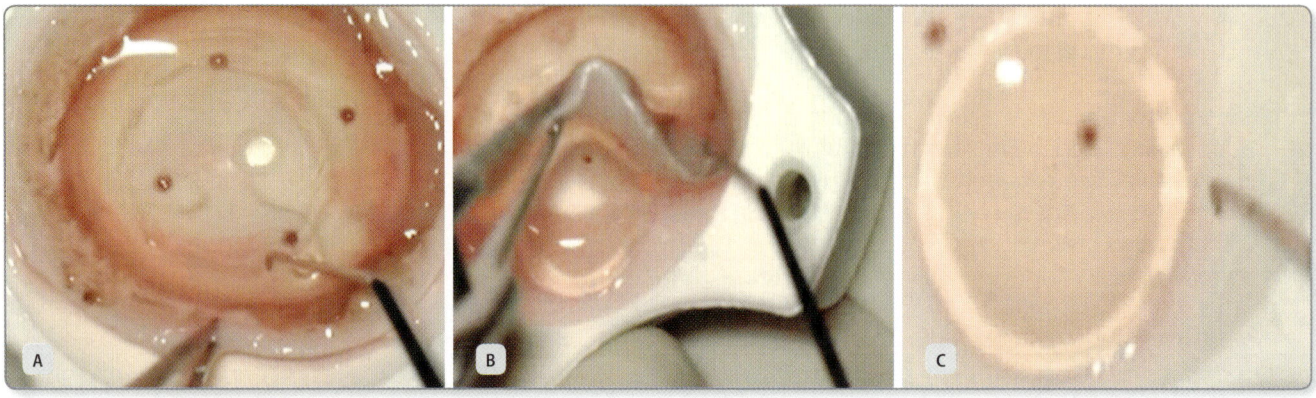

Figs 8.22A to C: The surgeon using an inverted Sinskey's hook that is able to separate the corneal lenticule from the sclerocorenal rim without needing a shrap instrument

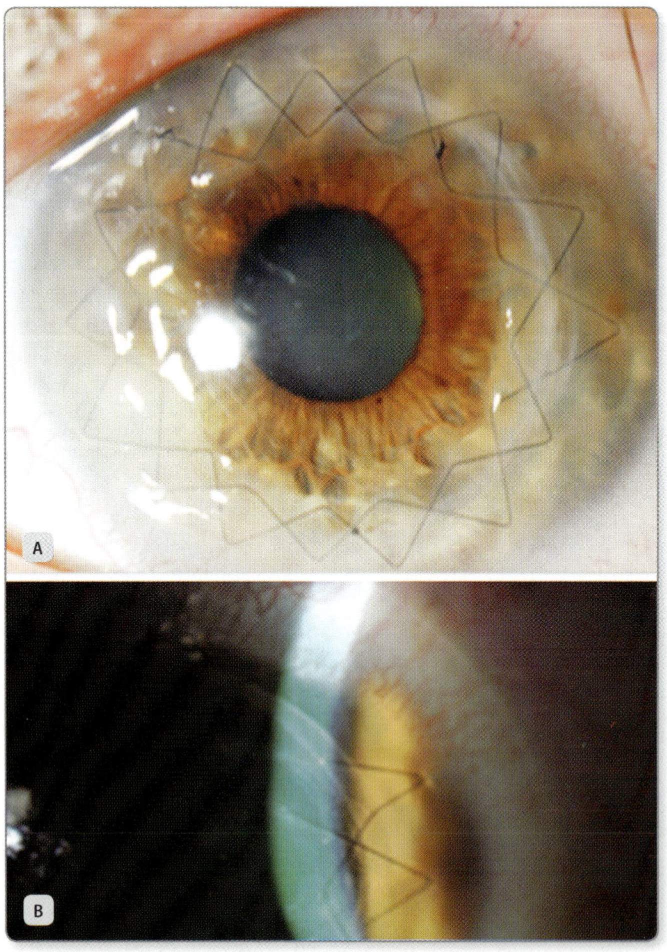

Figs 8.23A and B: Postoperative appearance of FSLAPKP

one *(P = 0.006)*, with 81% of the zig-zag group versus 45% of the conventional group were achieving BSCVA of more than or equal to 20/40 by the third month *(P = 0.03)* and this is similar to what have been published by Chamberlain et al.[12] and Gaster et al.[17] regarding the early significant difference in the early postoperative topographic astigmatism (Figs 8.24A and B).

Many authors published the higher stability of the top-hat pattern with higher wound leakage pressure,[11,15,17-20] but because of the larger posterior corneal tissue, which could increase the IOP and the possibility of endothelial rejection it has been investigated for other patterns to achieve better outcome with less complications.[21,22]

Optical coherence tomography examinations reveal no wound dehiscence and excellent appearance of graft-host tissue apposition and confirm that FSLAPKP offers benefits of rapid wound healing and predictable wound geometry.[23] We analyzed 11 eyes operated by FSLAPKP with different patterns (Mushroom, Zig-Zag and Top-Hat) using high-resolution (HR) anterior segment OCT (AS-OCT) to evaluate the posterior donor-host interface elevation (nasal and temporal sides) and the wound analysis of the zig-zag pattern reveals highly coopted donor-host interface in comparison to the mushroom and top-hat patterns **(**Figs 8.25A to C**)**.

The quality of vision, contrast sensitivity and higher orders aberration analysis were reported with favorable results using FSLAPKP[24,25] (Fig. 8.26).

Regarding the ultrastructure and microbiological studies, it was published that the femtosecond laser preserves the ultrastructure of the disrupted corneal collagen fibers,[26] prompts initial increase in keratocyte activation and dendritic cells that decrease over time,[27] favors corneal reinnervation as early as 1 month postoperatively[27] and does not increase the prevalence of positive microbiologic results or clinical infection.[28]

The few limitations for the femtosecond laser in PKP include difficulty to cut in peripheral corneal opacity and difficulty to achieve the desired planar cuts in eyes with significant anterior and posterior surface irregularities like Descemetocele[29] which can be overcome by optimization and innovations of the femtosecond technology.

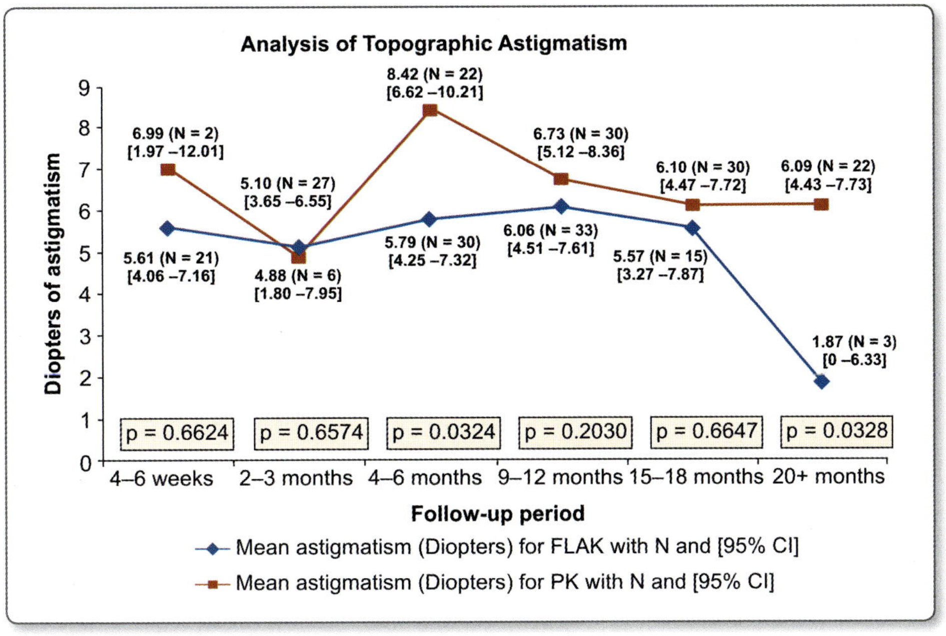

Fig. 8.24A: Analysis of topographic astigmatism: The mean astigmatism values for FSLAPKP) and conventional PKP at designated follow-up time points are shown in the graph. Means (calculated from the average of topographic simulated keratometry) are numerically depicted next to each data point with total number of subjects (N) in parentheses and confidence intervals (CI) in brackets. P-values generated from comparison of FSLAPKP versus PKP are shown at bottom of graph for each follow-up time point[12]

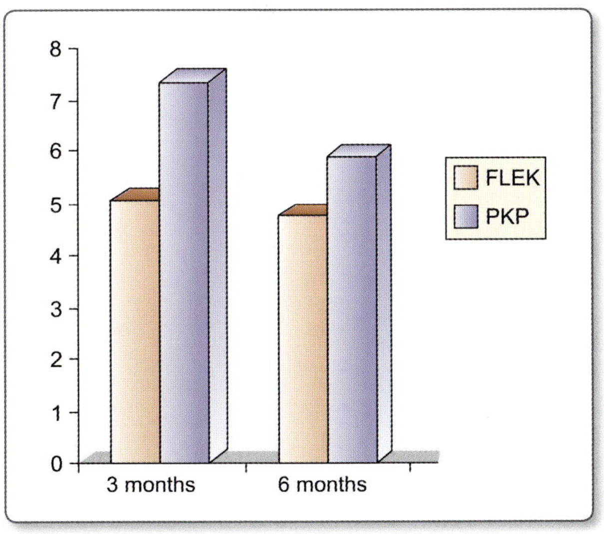

Fig. 8.24B: Time dynamic of topographically determined astigmatism (diopters) (p¼0.001)

Abbreviations: FLEK, femtosecond laser-enabled keratoplasty; PKP, penetrating keratoplasty.[17]

Cases Examples

Case 1

Figure 8.27A correspond to a male patient of 68-year-old that 20 years ago underwent phakic IOL implantation on his left eye. He presented to Vissum, Alicante ophthalmologic center with a visual acuity of 0.2 accompanied by corneal decompensation. Penetrating keratoplasty was the indication for surgery and a zig-zag pattern was the election. Figure 8.27B shows the postoperative results.

Case 2

Figures 8.28A and B correspond to a male patient of 78-year-old that came to our clinic with a corneal decompensation following a phacoemulsification procedure done 5 years ago. After the ophthalmological examination, it was decided to perform a FSLAPKP procedure. Penetrating keratoplasty was the indication for surgery and a zig-zag pattern was the election. Figures 8.28C shows the postoperative results.

CONCLUSIONS

Cornea transplant surgery has had a slow development in comparison to other ophthalmological procedures. The delicate tissue and what the cornea cicatrization represents for the rest of the optical system has not allow this development.

One of the most important improvements in the last decade, in corneal transplant has been the introduction of femtosecond laser technology. This technology has a great

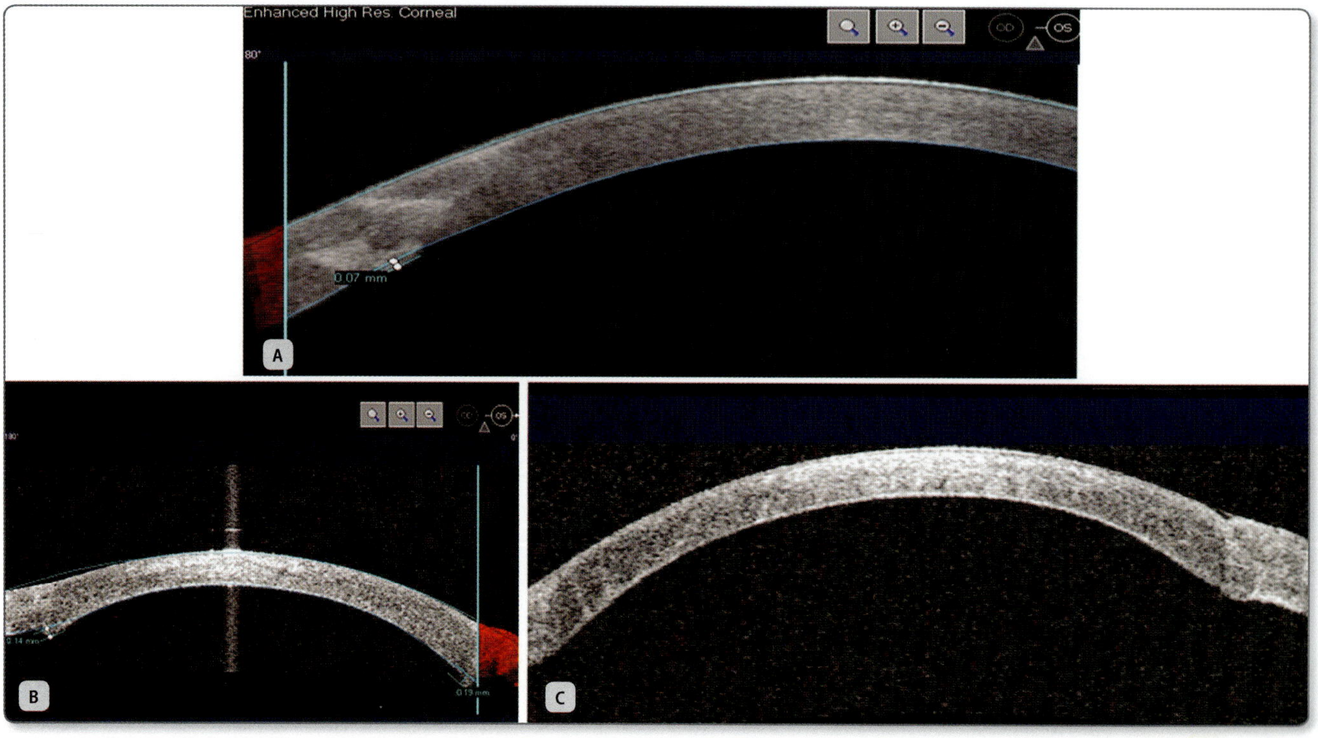

Figs 8.25A to C: Anterior segment OCT of FSLAPKP [(A) Zig-zag pattern (B) Mushroom-hat pattern and (C) Top-hat pattern]

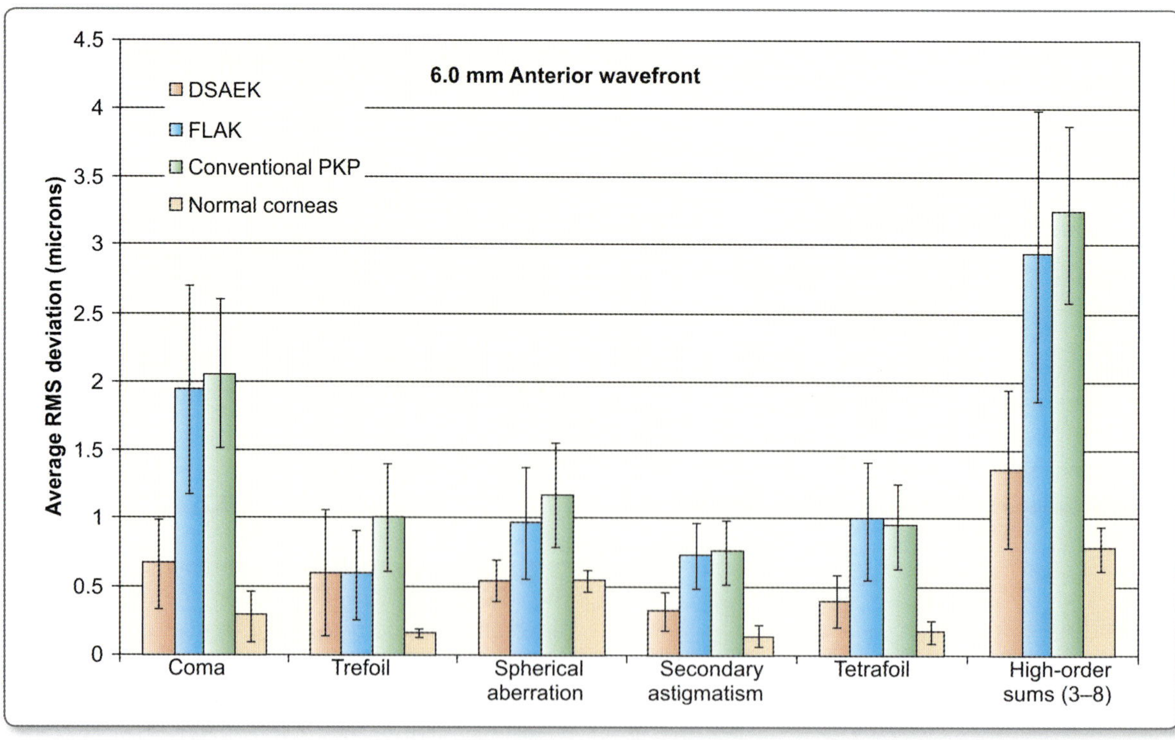

Fig. 8.26: Anterior corneal higher-order aberrations (HOAs) measured in in a 6.0-mm optical zone for post-Descemet's stripping automated endothelial keratoplasty (post-DSAEK), post-FSLAPKP, conventional post-PKP, and normal age matched corneas. Error bars represent standard deviation (SDs) for each group distribution[25]

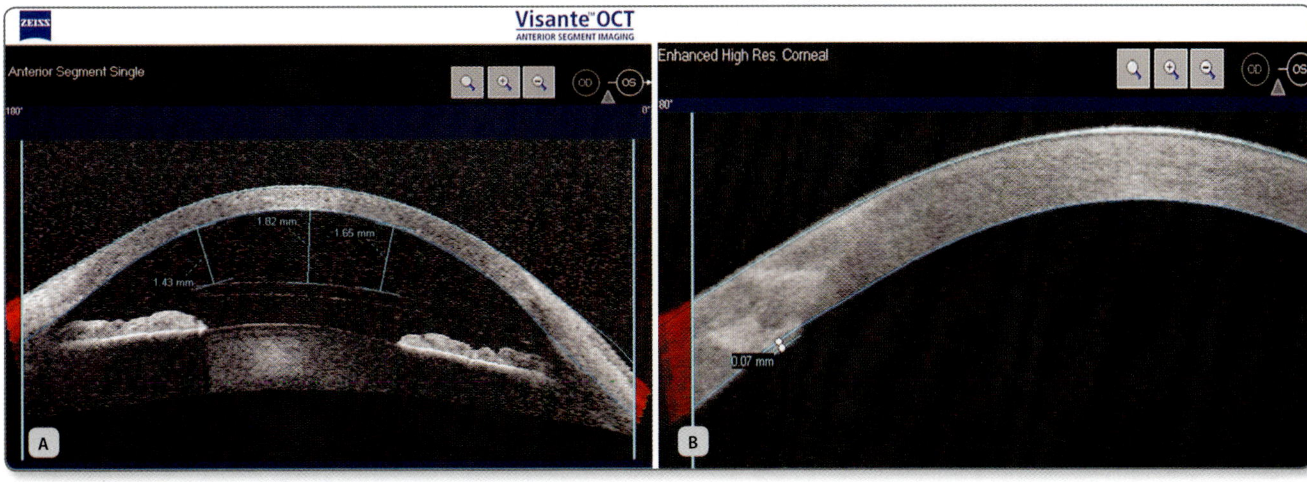

Figs 27A and B: Case 1: (A**)** Preoperative OCT image showing the distances below the safety margins between the phakic IOL and the endothelium before the femtosecond assisted PKP procedure; (B) The same patient 1 month after the surgical procedure. The white hyper-reflective line corresponds to the interface between the recipient and the donor tissue

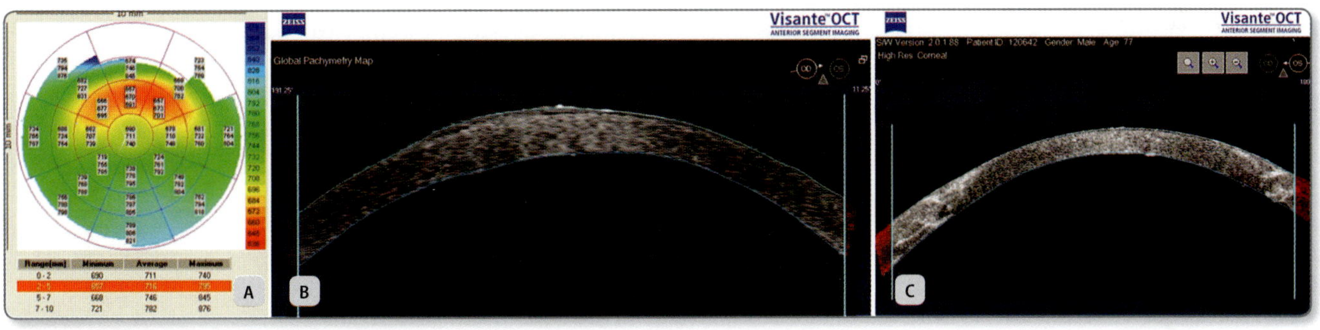

Figs 8.28A to C: Case 2: (A) Preoperative pachymetry image showing the cornea of a patient with corneal decompensation following a phacoemulsification procedure, (B) Preoperative OCT image showing a corneal edema with endothelial alteration morphology and (C) One month postoperative OCT image after a PKP procedure with a zig-zag pattern

acceptance among corneal surgeons because from the surgical standpoint is an intuitive technology, easy to learn and capable of improving the results based on it's perfect cut, giving excellent wound apposition and minimizing the suture tension depending of the pattern chosen. However, this technology is not meant to neglect the skills and training of surgeons, we believe that on the contrary is a technology where the manual procedure remains the most important piece in transplant surgery. Femtosecond technology allows in this moment the best decision to achieve the following goals:

- Excellent wound apposition
- Biomechanical stable incision
- Minimal suture with nominal voltage induced astigmatism
- Rapid recovery of the wound and vision
- Good selection of the incision type.

Despite of all the advantages that femtosecond laser has added to keratoplasty procedures there are still some improvements that have to be done in order to achieve an adequate technique that offers to the patients the best results in terms of functionality and refractive outcomes.

REFERENCES

1. Reinhart WJ, Musch DC, Jacobs DS, et al. Deep anterior lamellar keratoplasty as an alternative to penetrating keratoplasty: a report by the American Academy of Ophthalmology. Ophthalmol. 2011;118(1):209-18.
2. Richard JM, Paton D, Gasset AR. A comparison of penetrating keratoplasty and lamellar keratoplasty in the surgical management of keratoconus. Am J Ophthalmol. 1978;86(6):807-11.
3 Maier P, Böhringer D, Birnbaum F, et al. Improved wound stability of top-hat profiled femtosecond laser-assisted penetrating keratoplasty in vitro. Cornea. 2012;31(8):963-6.
4. Farid M, Kim M, Steinert RF. Results of penetrating keratoplasty performed with a femtosecond laser zig-zag incision initial report. Ophthalmol. 2007;114(12):2208-12.

5. Yoo SH, Hurmeric V. Femtosecond laser-assisted keratoplasty. Am J Ophthalmol. 2011;151(2):189-91.
6. Barraquer JI Jr. Technique of penetrating keratoplasty. Am J Ophthalmol. 1950;33(3 Pt 2):6-17.
7. Busin M. A new lamellar wound configuration for penetrating keratoplasty surgery. Arch Ophthalmol. 2003;121(2):260-5.
8. Gaster RN, Dumitrascu O, Rabinowitz YS. Penetrating keratoplasty using femtosecond laser-enabled keratoplasty with zig-zag incisions versus a mechanical trephine in patients with keratoconus. Br J Ophthalmol. 2012;96(9):1195-9.
9. Faktorovich E. Femtodynamics: a guide to laser settings and procedure techniques to optimize outcomes. Int Ophthalmol Clin. 2008;48(1):41-50.
10. Lahners WJ, Culbertson W, Rabinowitz Y, Azar D, Stahl J. (Eds). Femtosecond Laser in Corneal and Refractive Surgery. Online Interactive Ophthalmology Textbook. San Francisco, CA: American Academy of Ophthalmology. 2007.
11. Steinert RF, Ignacio TS, Sarayba MA. "Top-hat"-shaped penetrating keratoplasty using the femtosecond laser. Am J Ophthalmol. 2007;143(4):689-91.
12. Chamberlain WD, Rush SW, Mathers WD, et al. Comparison of femtosecond laser-assisted keratoplasty versus conventional penetrating keratoplasty. Ophthalmol. 2011;118(3):486-91.
13. Rush SW, Fraunfelder FW, Mathers WD, et al. Femtosecond laser-assisted keratoplasty in failed penetrating keratoplasty and globe trauma. Cornea. 2011;30(12):1358-62.
14. Graef S, Maier P, Boehringer D, et al. Femtosecond laser-assisted repeat keratoplasty: a case series. Cornea. 2011;30(6):687-91.
15. Bahar I, Kaiserman I, McAllum P, et al. Femtosecond laser-assisted penetrating keratoplasty: stability evaluation of different wound configurations. Cornea. 2008;27(2):209-11.
16. Farid M, Steinert RF, Gaster RN, et al. Comparison of penetrating keratoplasty performed with a femtosecond laser zig-zag incision versus conventional blade trephination. Ophthalmol. 2009;116(9):1638-43.
17. Gaster RN, Dumitrascu O, Rabinowitz YS. Penetrating keratoplasty using femtosecond laser-enabled keratoplasty with zig-zag incisions versus a mechanical trephine in patients with keratoconus. Br J Ophthalmol. 2012;96(9):1195-9.
18. Ignacio TS, Nguyen TB, Chuck RS, et al. Top-hat wound configuration for penetrating keratoplasty using the femtosecond laser: a laboratory model. Cornea. 2006;25(3):336-40.
19. Maier P, Böhringer D, Birnbaum F, et al. Improved wound stability of top-hat profiled femtosecond laser-assisted penetrating keratoplasty in vitro. Cornea. 2012;31(8):963-6.
20. Birnbaum F, Wiggermann A, Maier PC, et al. Clinical results of 123 femtosecond laser-assisted penetrating keratoplasties. Graefes Arch Clin Exp Ophthalmol. 2013;251(1):95-103.
21. Fung SS, Iovieno A, Shanmuganathan VA, et al. Femtosecond laser-assisted lock-and-key shaped penetrating keratoplasty. Br J Ophthalmol. 2012;96(1):136-7.
22. Gilmer W, McLeod SD, Jeng BH. Laboratory model of bursting pressures of femtosecond laser-assisted penetrating keratoplasty wounds using novel pattern designs. Br J Ophthalmol. 2012;96(9):1273-4.
23. Heur M, Tang M, Yiu S, et al. Investigation of femtosecond laser-enabled keratoplasty wound geometry using optical coherence tomography. Cornea. 2011;30(8):889-94.
24. Cheng YY, van den Berg TJ, Schouten JS, Pels E, Wijdh RJ, van Cleynenbreugel H, et al. Quality of vision after femtosecond laser-assisted descemet stripping endothelial keratoplasty and penetrating keratoplasty: a randomized, multicenter clinical trial. Am J Ophthalmol. 2011;152(4):556-66.
25. Chamberlain W, Omid N, Lin A, et al. Comparison of corneal surface higher-order aberrations after endothelial keratoplasty, femtosecond laser-assisted keratoplasty, and conventional penetrating keratoplasty. Cornea. 2012;31(1):6-13.
26. Nuzzo V, Aptel F, Savoldelli M, et al. Histologic and ultrastructural characterization of corneal femtosecond laser trephination. Cornea. 2009;28(8):908-13.
27. Shtein RM, Kelley KH, Musch DC, et al. In vivo confocal microscopic evaluation of corneal wound healing after femtosecond laser-assisted keratoplasty. Ophthalmic Surg Lasers Imaging. 2012;43(3):205-13.
28. Garg S, Said B, Farid M, et al. Prevalence of positive microbiology results from donor cornea tissue in different methods of corneal transplantation. Cornea. 2013;32(2):137-40.
29. Yoo SH, Hurmeric V. Femtosecond laser-assisted keratoplasty. Am J Ophthalmol. 2011;151(2):189-91.

Chapter

9

Femtosecond Laser-Assisted Anterior Lamellar Keratoplasty (FLALK) with IntraLase Technology (Use of the Different Technologies, Surgical Practical Pearls, Outcomes)

Jorge L Alió, Alfredo Vega, Felipe Soria, Ahmed A Abdou

CHAPTER OUTLINE

- Preoperative considerations when deciding femtosecond (FS) assisted anterior lamellar graft surgery
  - Indications
  - Preoperative evaluation
  - General considerations
  - Anesthesia
  - Ophthalmological examination
- Surgical procedure for corneal receptor; selection of the sidecut profile; Usefulness of the big-bubble technique in the dissection of the deep stroma
- Surgical procedure for corneal donor with the Moria's artificial anterior chamber (AAC)
- Practical considerations when performing the surgery and suturing technique
- Overview of the outcomes reported in deep anterior lamellar keratoplasty (DALK) assisted by FS technology

INTRODUCTION

The first documented penetrating keratoplasty (PK) in humans was performed by Eduard Zirm in 1905.[1] Another pioneer in this surgical technique was Ramon Castroviejo who improved the technique of the operation in the 30s and 40s, prompting the worldwide adoption of corneal transplantation as a standard until more efficient suture materials became available.[2] Since then, this surgical procedure has evolved significantly, thanks to the advance in the technology of the different tools that are used. Nevertheless, rejection of the donor tissue is still the main complication and disadvantages of full lamellar techniques, which is mediated primarily by immunological response against corneal endothelial cells.[3]

On the other hand, lamellar keratoplasty (LK) is a technique whereby a partial-thickness corneal transplant is performed for various indications in order to avoid the potential complications observed when performing PK.[1] The first corneal transplant was performed in the 19th century by Von Hippel and it was a lamellar procedure.[3] Afterwards, several ophthalmic surgeons including Filatov in the 30s, Paufique in the 40s, Barraquer in the 50s and others have developed and used LK as an alternative to PK for the treatment of corneal disease.[4] However, most of these investigators found very poor visual outcomes due to irregularity of the dissected surfaces and scaring of the interfaces.[4] During the decade of 70s, Gasset carried out an investigation with keratoconus patients in which he transplanted a corneal graft without Descemet's membrane (DM) into a deep lamellar bed recipient.[5] Since then, several surgical techniques have been developed in order to remove the corneal stroma, leaving the DM of the corneal recipient with the aim of treating corneal pathologies with normal endothelium, procedure that is nowadays worldwide known as deep anterior lamellar keratoplasty (DALK).

Many maneuvers have been described in order to bare the DM in DALK procedures. Sugita and Kondo first introduced a hydro-delamination technique where they used fluid in order to separate the DM.[6] Another approach was described by Melles in which he performed the dissection of the DM from the corneal stroma by using ophthalmic viscosurgical device.[7] One of the techniques that is more spread among ophthalmic surgeons is the "Big-bubble" technique. This maneuver was described by Anwar and Teichmann in which the dissection of the DM from the corneal stroma is achieved by means of an injection of air into the deep stroma that greatly facilitates the removal of the remaining tissue in the trephine bed.[8]

Nowadays, with the introduction of the femtosecond (FS) laser in ophthalmic surgery, DALK procedures have taken a big step in the daily practice of the ophthalmologist. Outcomes of FS assisted keratoplasty have demonstrated an improvement in terms of visual recovery and reduction of corneal astigmatism in comparison with other keratoplasty procedures.[9] In addition, the different patterns that can be performed with the FS allow an excellent apposition of the tissue that results in a rapid wound healing, which will lead to more earlier removal of the suture and a faster recovery of the patients.[10]

In this chapter we will present to the reader some pearls that we have learned from our own experience after many years of practicing and improving our FS DALK procedures. We hope that in the oncoming lines, the surgeon and the surgical team can find the tools that will lead them to a better management and development, the expertise for improving their FS DALK procedures.

FEMTOSECOND LASER-ASSISTED DEEP ANTERIOR LAMELLAR KERATOPLASTY

Preoperative Considerations

Indications

The main indications for FSDALK procedure will be those cases in which there is a corneal disease with normal DM and corneal endothelium such as:

- *Corneal ectasia*: Keratoconus is by far the most common indication of DALK procedure. We have to take into account that the patient should not have a history of corneal hydrops in which case DALK has to be considered as a contraindication due to the rupture of the DM. Other pathologies that enter into this group are pellucid marginal degeneration and post-laser-assisted in situ keratomileusis (LASIK) ectasia.
- *Corneal dystrophies*
- *Corneal scars* due to trauma or infectious keratitis

Preoperative Evaluation

As the main objective of this procedure is to re-establish the best visual acuity possible, the clinician must perform a complete ophthalmological evaluation having the absolute certainty of the potential vision of the patient. We usually indicate DALK procedures in those patients in which their best spectacle corrected vision is worse than 0.2 in the decimal notation, the patient is not tolerant to wear contact lenses and when other treatments such as intracorneal ring segments have failed or are contraindicated. On the other hand, the clinician must explain to the patient about the expectations in terms of the visual acuity that the patient will achieve after the surgery and also to take into consideration the possible complications and the fact of a prolonged postoperative treatment. The patients must know that they will reach their complete visual potential after the sutures are removed and a refractive treatment is instituted and this usually will take at least 6 months, in this way the patient would not have false expectations or be frustrated by the visual acuity achieved in the immediate postoperative period.

General Considerations

Usually, patients that undergo this type of procedure are young and do not require consultation by the intern medicine or the anesthesiologist department. However, exploration about bleeding disorders and related drugs must be recognized. Patients receiving anticoagulants are advised to cease 7 days before the surgery, the intake of their medication because of the increased risk of bleeding during the surgery. In case that a general anesthesia is indicated, the patient should undergo a full systemic evaluation preferably carried out by the internist or anesthesiologist.

Anesthesia[11]

(For detail see Chapter 8)

OPHTHALMOLOGICAL EXAMINATION

Visual Acuity and Refraction

In our experience, we usually indicate DALK procedures in those patients in which their best spectacle corrected vision is worse than 0.2 in the decimal notation, the patient is not tolerant to wear contact lenses and when other treatments such as intracorneal ring segments have failed or are contraindicated.

Corneal Topography

Although corneal topography may not be possible to perform because of severe irregularity of the anterior corneal surface, it is mandatory to do it in keratoconus cases to evaluate the conditions of the fellow eye. It may also be helpful to assess the presence of peripheral ectasia and cases of pellucid marginal degeneration.

Corneal Pachymetry

The best way to evaluate the panoramic thickness of the corneal tissue is by means of a corneal pachymetry map (Fig. 9.1). A pachymetry map will allow us to assess the precise thickness of the cornea where the FS will pass through them. Measuring the central and peripheral corneal thickness will allow us to determine the parameters of the incisions for our surgical planning. A pachymetry map can be performed with both, ultrasound pachymetry and optical coherence tomography (OCT). In our practice, we prefer the second method as it gives us a more detailed thickness within 10 mm of corneal diameter.

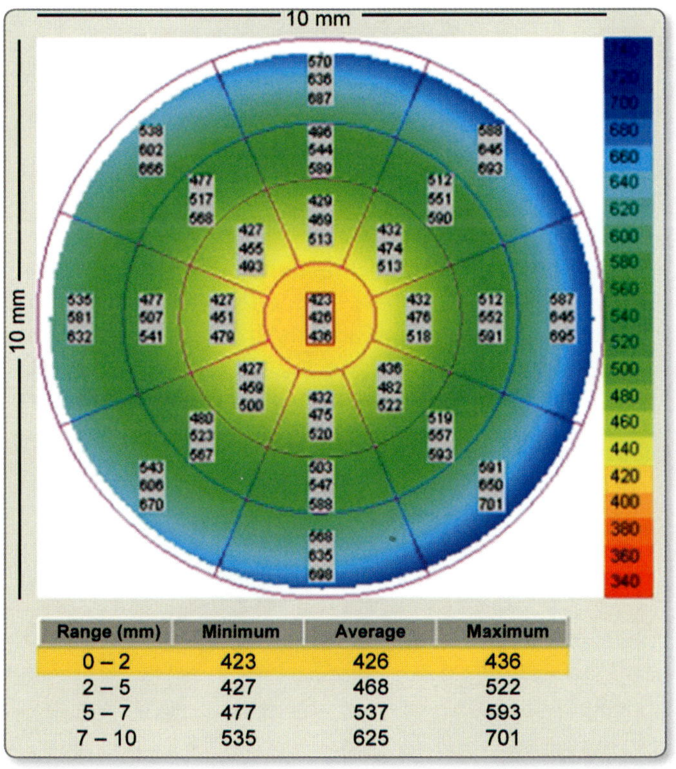

Range (mm)	Minimum	Average	Maximum
0 – 2	423	426	436
2 – 5	427	468	522
5 – 7	477	537	593
7 – 10	535	625	701

Fig. 9.1: The pachymetry map of a keratoconus patient that will undergo femtosecond (FS) assisted deep anterior lamellar keratoplasty (DALK) surgery

Anterior Segment Optical Coherence Tomography

The anterior segment OCT is a very important tool that will allow us to perform not only a corneal pachymetry map, but also an evaluation of the anatomy of the anterior chamber from the iris until the posterior surface of the cornea. It is also important to note the OCT capacity to obtain the dimensions (depth and longitude) of the opacities in the cornea and evaluate the possibility of FS to break through them (see Fig. 8.3). In our experience, we suggest not to perform the FS for the dissection of the cornea when the thickness is below 350 µm because of overlapping of the incisions.

Specular Microscopy

Evaluation of the corneal endothelium is mandatory when planning a DALK procedure. As most of the patients undergoing DALK are young patients, usually the endothelial cell count is within normal levels. However, we have to be aware that in case low endothelial cell density a penetrating procedure should be indicated.

SURGICAL PROCEDURE FOR CORNEAL RECEPTOR

Femtosecond technology allows us to perform different staggered patterns that otherwise cannot be achieved with a standard corneal trephine. These designs will result in an excellent apposition of the tissue, which will lead to a rapid wound healing and an earlier removal of the suture with a faster recovery of the patients.

Even though IntraLase technology let us perform three different types of corneal pattern incisions, in our experience we prefer to do a "mushroom pattern" when we are performing DALK procedures.

We describe below the settings that we introduce in the IntraLase in order to perform the "mushroom pattern" as well as the benefits and disadvantages that we have encountered with this technique:

Mushroom Pattern (Figs 9.2A and B)

Benefits

Larger amounts of corneal tissue are added to the thin periphery and minimize the extraction of healthy endothelium.

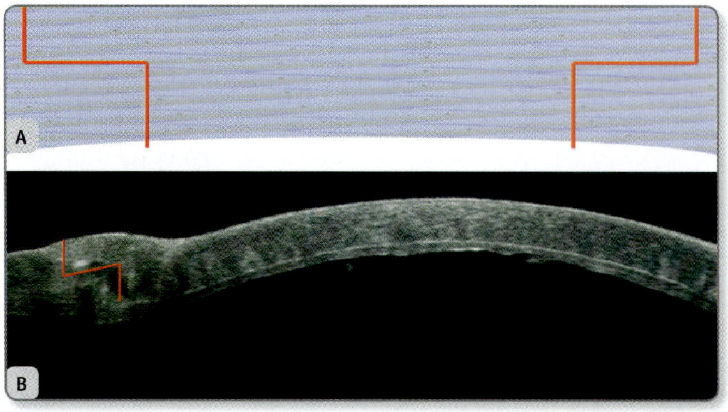

Figs 9.2A and B: (A) Schematic view of the "mushroom" pattern as created by the IntraLase; (B) 1 week postoperative optical coherence tomography (OCT) image of the cornea of a patient that underwent deep anterior lamellar keratoplasty (DALK); Red lines show the mushroom pattern created by the IntraLase in this case

Disadvantages

The straight-edge-to-straight-edge configuration is associated with delayed, weak and incomplete healing of the donor-host junction.

IntraLase Settings Sample

Ring lamellar cut:	On
Depth in cornea:	280
Outer diameter:	8.5
Inner diameter:	7.5
Energy:	1.90
Tangential spot separation:	4
Radial spot separation:	4
Spiral start:	Out
Full lamellar cut:	Off
Anterior side cut:	On
Posterior depth:	300
Anterior diameter:	8.4
Energy:	2.05
Cut position 1:	0
Cut angle 1:	360
Cut position 2:	180
Cut angle 2:	0
Anterior side cut angle:	90
Anterior side cut spot separation:	3
Anterior side cut layer separation:	2
Depth in glass:	50
Posterior side cut:	On
Anterior depth:	260
Posterior diameter:	7.6
Posterior energy:	2.05
Posterior post depth:	
Thinnest pachymetry point:	125 µm
70% of the thinnest pachymetry point	
Posterior side cut angle:	90
Posterior side cut spot separation:	3
Posterior side cut layer separation:	2
Alignment incisions:	Off

When all the settings are rationally established in the IntraLase by the assistant, double check by the surgeon and the patient is lying in the couch, their routine approach is the following:

- Select the optical wheel of the IntraLase to position D and focus on the receptor cornea.
- Verify with a caliper the white-to-white measurement (Fig. 9.3). This will allow assessing, if the diameter that was programmed in the FS parameters is in concordance with the diameter of the cornea. It also helps to make sure that the dissection of the FS will be outside of the intracorneal ring segments in case that those were previously implanted.
- Ultrasonic pachymetry measurements in situ in order to make sure that the values correspond to those previously measured by OCT (Fig. 9.4).
  Starting in the center and placing the probe in the intended zone of the incisions, approximately in the midperiphery of the cardinal points following the midperiphery obliquely to the cardinal points (between 7 mm and 9 mm), in total, the authors suggest at least nine measurements. This data should be compared with the OCT pachymetry.
- With a marker, proceed to check the center of the cornea for an accurate centration of the dissection with the FS (Fig. 9.5).
- Eye fixation with corneal suction ring (Fig. 9.6).
  The easiest way to achieve a good suction of the eye ball is to have the assistant hold the inferior eye lid, and the surgeon will hold the upper lid, the inferior border of the

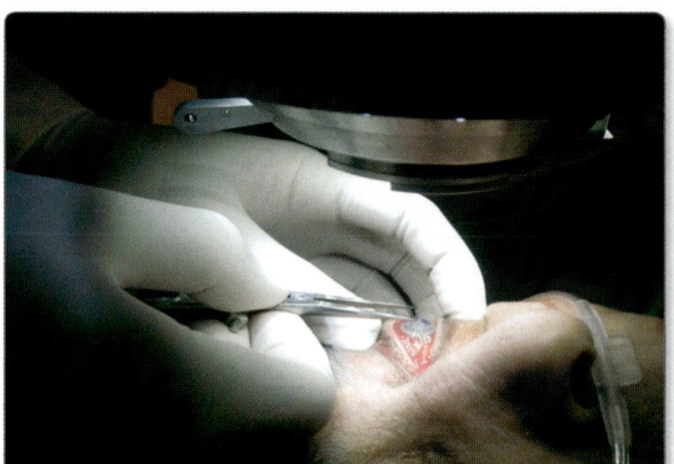

Fig. 9.3: The measurement of the white-to-white distances in order to plan the diameter of the dissection with the IntraLase

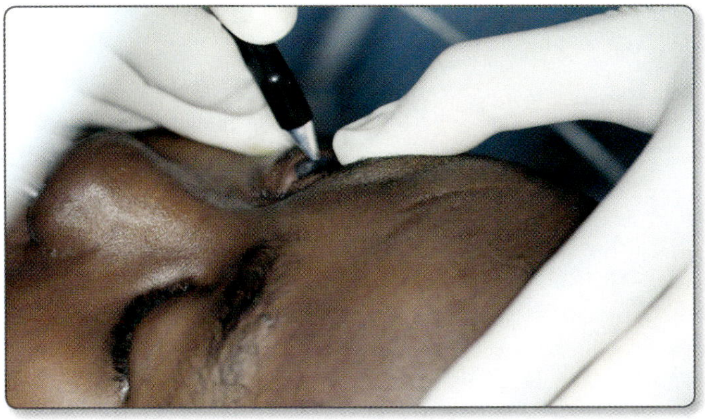

Fig. 9.4: The ultrasonic pachymetry in situ to double check the pachymetry map previously performed with the help of optical coherence tomography (OCT)

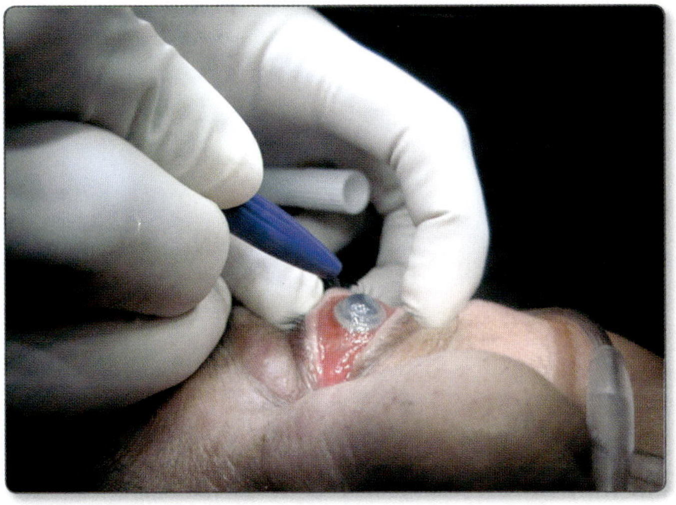

Fig. 9.5: The method to mark the center of the cornea in order to assess a better centration of the femtosecond (FS) dissection

ring will gently but firmly placed over the inferior globe; after this, the ring will be placed over the sclera, making sure to achieve the best symmetrical position. As soon the best position is achieved, suction will be demanded.

- Cone positioning and perpendicular docking (Fig. 9.7). One of the most important steps in this procedure is to achieve a perfect docking. When lowering down the cone, the optical wheel will be changed to position 2 and the key orientation will be the circular light pattern of the illumination mechanism projected over the cornea. We suggest to always call these step perpendicular docking, because we emphasize in the surgeons mind the correct positioning of the cone over the cornea. When contact is made with the cornea, a meniscus will be seen starting from the center and moving to the periphery in an equal way. If the meniscus is not even, gently corrections can be made to the side moving the suction ring where the meniscus is greater, but "never" the joystick in the X/Y direction. When the meniscus left behind the cutting pattern, the clip can be opened (Figs 9.8A and B).
- Centration of the dissection. After the suction ring is fixated into the eye globe, the assistant will center the dissection circle from the screen of the IntraLase on the mark that was previously done by the surgeon in the cornea (Fig. 9.9).
- *Pressing the foot pedal*: During this step, it is essential that all personnel in the operating room (OR) stand still making sure that no one touches the operating table or the IntraLase. Also assure that all cell phones are off.
  - *Normal view*: Depending on the patterns, the laser always starts the cuts from posterior to anterior, so what the surgeon must see is the presence of the bubbles generated by the laser in the deep stroma.
  - *Abnormal view*:
    - *Bubbles in anterior chamber*: If at the moment when the foot pedal is pressed, the surgeons notice the presence of bubbles in the anterior

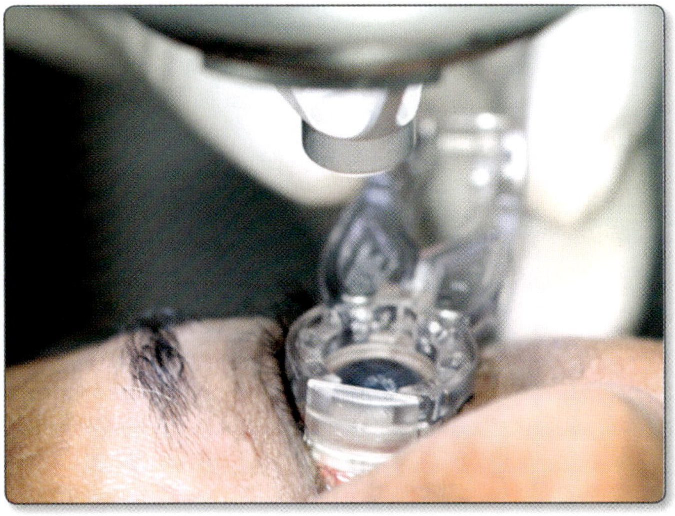

Fig. 9.6: Eye fixation with the suction ring just before performing the dissection with the IntraLase

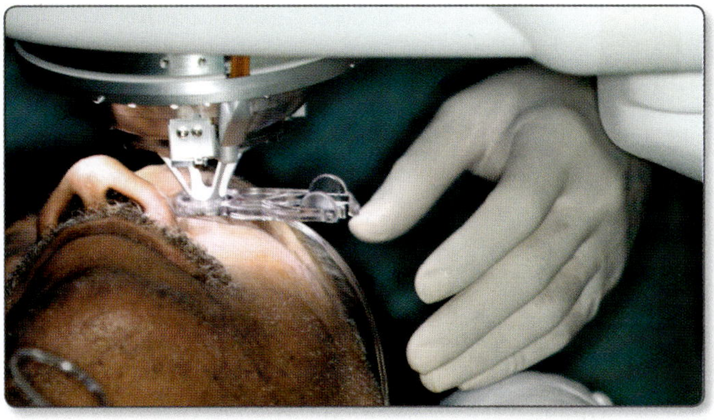

Fig. 9.7: The moment of the perpendicular docking

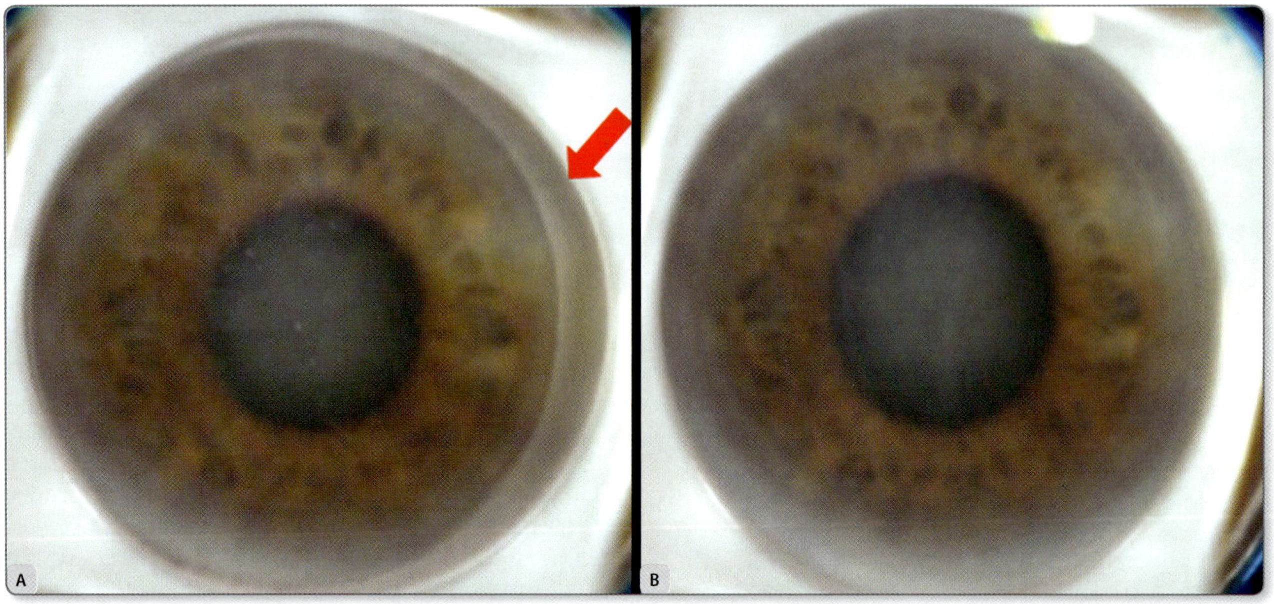

Figs 9.8A and B: (A) An uneven docking lies with the presence of meniscus in the right side of the image (solid red arrow). (B) An adequate docking with complete absence of meniscus and the green light "on", which means that the IntraLase system is ready to start with the dissection

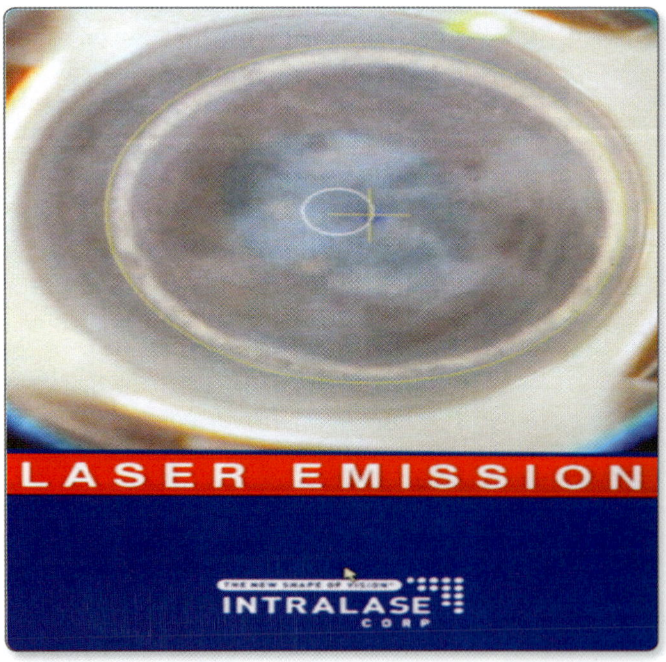

Fig. 9.9: Centering the dissection on the mark previously done in the center of the cornea

chamber; the procedure should be aborted and new settings of the parameter changing the depth of the posterior side cut should be performed.

- The eye is patched and then the patient is transferred to a stretcher and taken to the OR where the procedure will be completed. In our settings, this is easy, safe and fast because we have a door leading directly to the OR. Ideally the surgical extraction of the cornea receptor starts meanwhile the donor cornea procedure has been done. Experience allows us to do both procedures parallel and when the surgeon requires the donor cornea these one will be ready.
- Some key features that the surgeon should have taken into account are that separating the tissue previously dissected with the FS can be achieved with a Sinskey's hook without needing a corneal trephine or knife. We suggest separating the cornea with the Sinskey's hook, all 360° beginning in the upper side of the pattern and then continue with the deeper side. Afterwards, using a Crescent knife, the surgeon will proceed to remove the anterior aspect of the corneal stroma parallel to the plane corresponding to the base of the "mushroom" (Figs 9.10A and B). Once this is performed, the surgeon will continue with his habitual standard DALK procedure.

SURGICAL PROCEDURE FOR CORNEAL DONOR WITH THE MORIA'S ARTIFICIAL ANTERIOR CHAMBER (FIG. 9.11)

During this procedure, the patient is kept in the OR where the recipient tissue is being removed. Ideally, perform this procedure before the surgeon begins with the surgery in the patient.

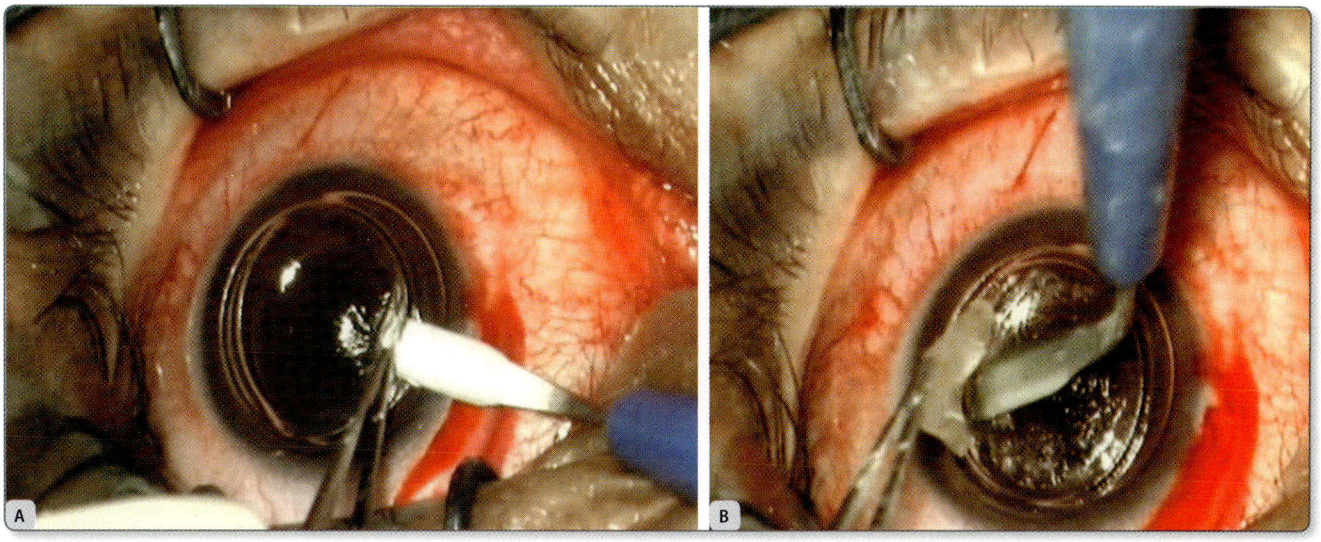

Figs 9.10A and B: The surgeon removing the anterior part of the stroma, which is parallel to the plane corresponding to the base of the "mushroom" with the help of Crescent knife

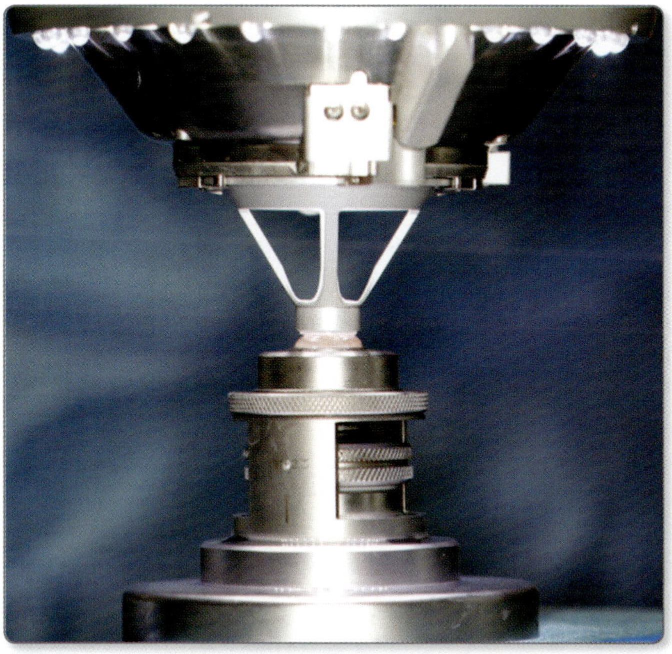

Fig. 9.11: Moria's artificial anterior chamber (AAC)

Setting up the Materials

Using aseptic technique, a table should be covered with a sterile field where the following instruments will be placed (see Fig. 8.13):

- Donor corneal tissue
- Medicine cup with 10 mL of chlorhexidine
- Medical cup with 50 mL of balanced salt solution (BSS)
- Artificial anterior chamber (AAC)
- Forceps
- Caliper
- Surgical sponge
- Barraquer's tonometer
- A 10 mL syringe

Setting up the Sclerocorneal Donor in the Anterior Artificial Chamber and Proceeding with the IntraLaser Procedure

The procedure begins with a 5 minutes surgical scrub technique followed by the placement of sterile gown and gloves.

- Connect the 10 mL syringe with the three-way stopcock of the AAC (Fig. 9.12).

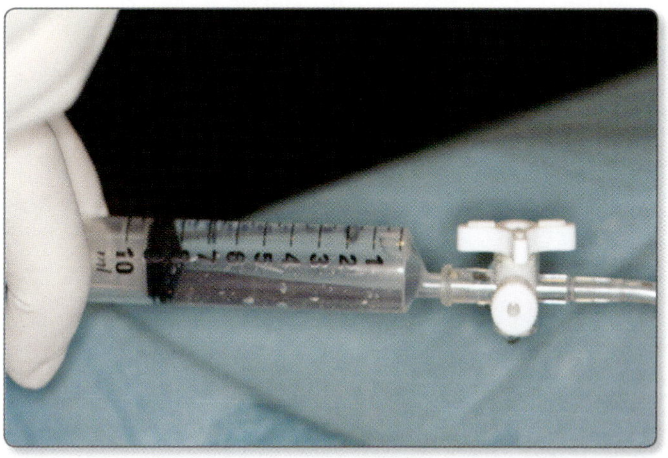

Fig. 9.12: Connecting the 10 mL syringe with the three-way stopcock of the artificial anterior chamber (AAC)

- Fill up the syringe with 10 mL of BSS and connect it to the Infusion intravenous (IV) line injecting BSS until the concave superior part of the piston is filled with BSS (Fig. 9.13A).
- Place the sclerocorneal donor graft on the piston with the endothelium facing down using the forceps. Achieve a good centration making sure that no sclera is over the concave part of the piston (Fig. 9.13B).
- Hold the graft with the forceps, and with the other hand, inject BBS in order to eliminate any air bubble. Gently movements of the graft can be done to achieve the elimination of air bubbles. When this is achieved, place the three-way stopcock in the position "closed" (Fig. 9.13C).
- Fit the anterior chamber cover over the graft and lock it in place with a 15° clockwise turn (Fig. 9.13D).
- Elevate the piston in order to tighten the chamber to the base and fixate the sclerocorneal rim (Fig. 9.13E).
- Measure the IOP with the Barraquer's tonometer to make sure that an adequate pressure is present in the sclerocorneal rim. (Fig. 9.13F).
- Place the table below the FS and using the same docking that was used in the cornea of the patient, thus the incisions must match precisely (Fig. 9.13G).
- Select the optical wheel of the IntraLase to position D and focus on the sclerocorneal rim (Fig. 9.13H).
- With a marker, proceed to mark the center of the cornea in order to achieve an adequate centration of the dissection (Fig. 9.13I).
- Make sure that the three-way stopcock is in position "closed".
- Cone positioning and perpendicular docking (Fig. 9.14).
- When placing down the cone, the optical wheel of the IntraLase will be changed to position 2 and the key orientation will be the circular light pattern of the illumination mechanism projected over the cornea. The authors suggest to always call these step perpendicular docking, because they emphasize in the surgeons mind the correct positioning of the cone. When contact is made with the cornea, ask the assistant in the IntraLase to center the dissection on the mark that was previously done by the surgeon. Sometimes, if a small bubble was left inside the AAC, like the one shown in Figure 9.15 the procedure can also be centered in the bubble as usually it will be found in the center of the endothelium side of the sclerocorneal rim. Finish the perpendicular docking until the meniscus is even or completely disappear. If the meniscus is not even, gently corrections can be made to the side where the meniscus is greater. When the meniscus is left behind and the green light is turned on, correct docking is achieved.
- Double check together with the assistant that the correct pattern was designed ("preview pattern" in the IntraLase) (Fig. 9.16).
- Pressing the foot pedal:
  - *Normal view*: Depending on the patterns, the laser always starts the cuts from posterior to anterior, so what the surgeon must see in the first instance is the formation of air bubbles inside the AAC.

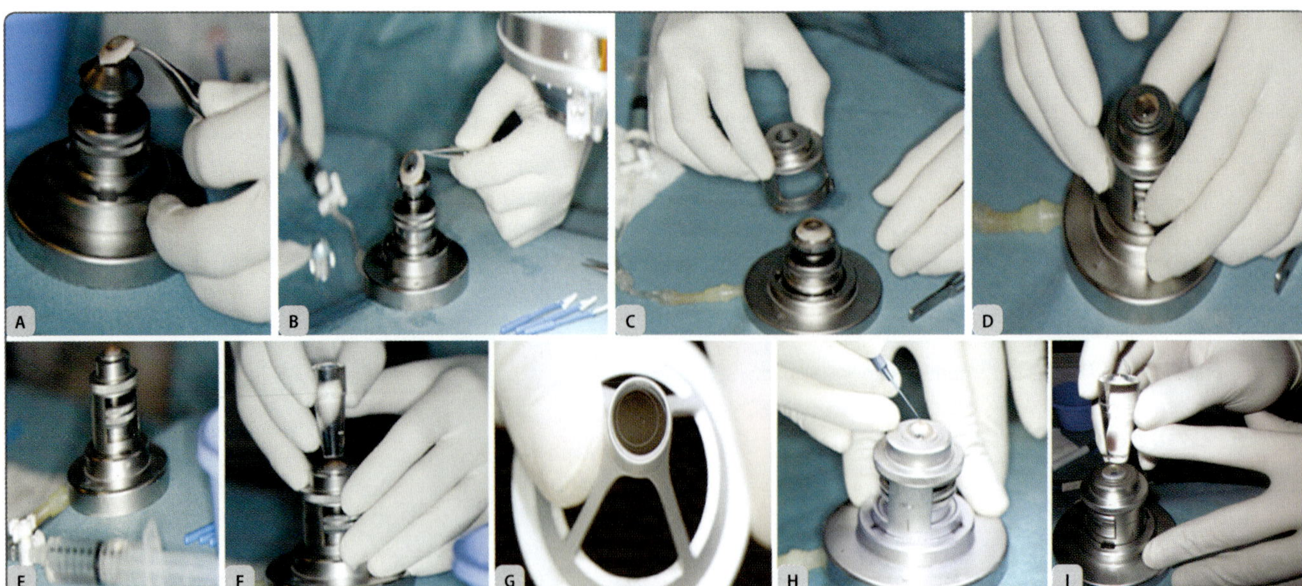

Figs 9.13A to I: Steps for an adequate placement of the donor cornea on the Moria's artificial anterior chamber (AAC); refer to the text for description of the image

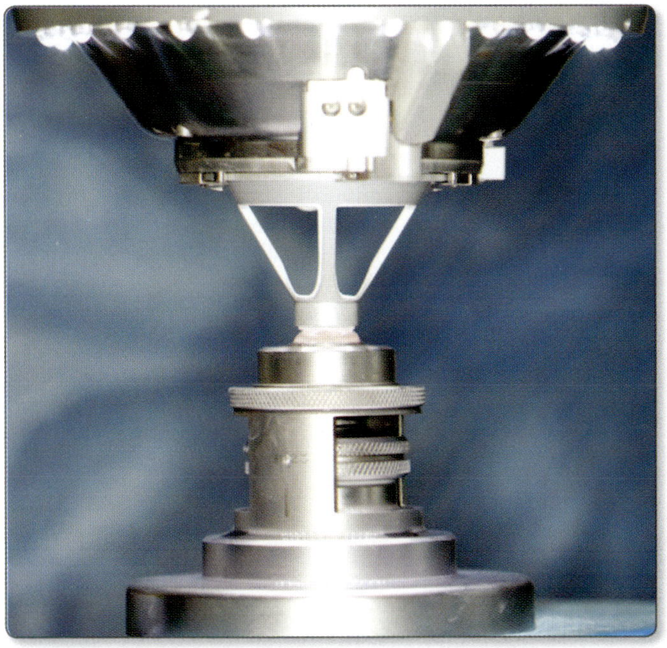

Fig. 9.14: Perpendicular docking on the donor graft

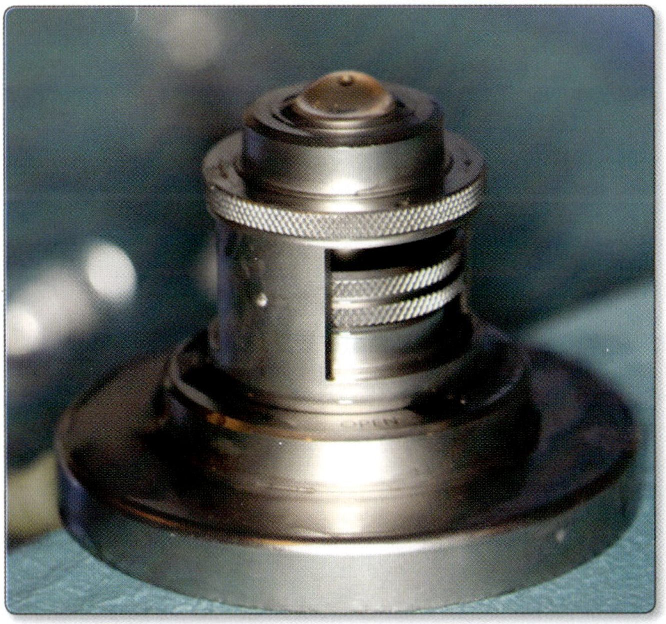

Fig. 9.15: The small bubble inside the artificial anterior chamber (AAC) that allows centering the dissection

- *Abnormal view*:
  - *Uneven dissection pattern*: The procedure should not be stopped but the surgeon must have in consideration that the part of the cornea that was not properly dissected will not be easily removed from the sclera.

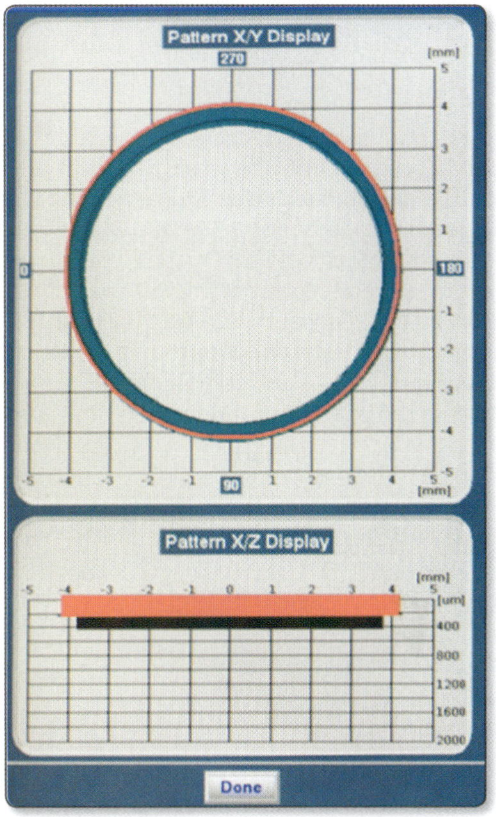

Fig. 9.16: Mushroom "preview pattern"

- The corneal graft is placed in the medical cap with chlorhexidine and is taken to the OR for the implantation.
- *Undocking*: The elevation of the cone should be done slowly to observe the behavior of the donor cornea. If it is observed that the cornea is collapsing, BSS must be injected.
- Releasing the anterior chamber cover requires of very slow movements, the same as when lowering the piston. Doing both of these steps requires concomitantly the injection of BSS thus the cornea does not collapse. This avoids the creation of striae and probably loss of endothelial cells.
- The corneal graft is placed in the medical cap with chlorhexidine and it is taken to the OR for its implantation.
- Once in the OR, the donor cornea can be dissected from the sclera rim by using an inverted Sinskey's hook. If an even dissection pattern was achieved with the FS, grasping the sclera rim with a forcep and dissecting with the inverted Sinskey's hook around the 360° of the incision with the sclerocorneal rim over the donor cap, should be enough to get the corneal lenticule away from the scleral rim (see Figs 8.22A to C). Afterwards, the surgeon will continue with his habitual standard DALK procedure.

Figures 9.17 and 9.18 illustrated two clinical cases of keratoconus patients that underwent DALK assisted by FS laser. Case 1 (Figs 9.17A and B) correspond to a female patient of 27 years old that was previously implanted with intracorneal ring segments on her left eye. The disease continued to progress until the visual acuity fall to 0.2 in the decimal scale and it was decided to perform a FS assisted DALK procedure. Case 2 (Figs 9.18A and B) correspond to a male patient of 21 years old that came to our clinic with an advance form of keratoconus on his left eye with corrected vision of 0.1 on the decimal scale. After the ophthalmological examination, it was decided to perform a FS assisted DALK procedure. Figures 9.18A and B show the OCT image of the cornea before the procedure and 2 weeks after the surgery.

OVERVIEW OF OUTCOMES REPORTED IN FEMTOSECOND ASSISTED DALK

There are several factors, which make difficult to carry out a proper analysis of the outcomes obtained after DALK procedure. The different methods of baring the DM, the technologies used to perform the dissection of the recipient and the donor tissue, the different suturing techniques, among others, have to be considered as factors that will impact in the results obtained by different authors. Nevertheless, we can get an insight of the outcomes after DALK procedure by analyzing the different scientific data that have been published over the last years.

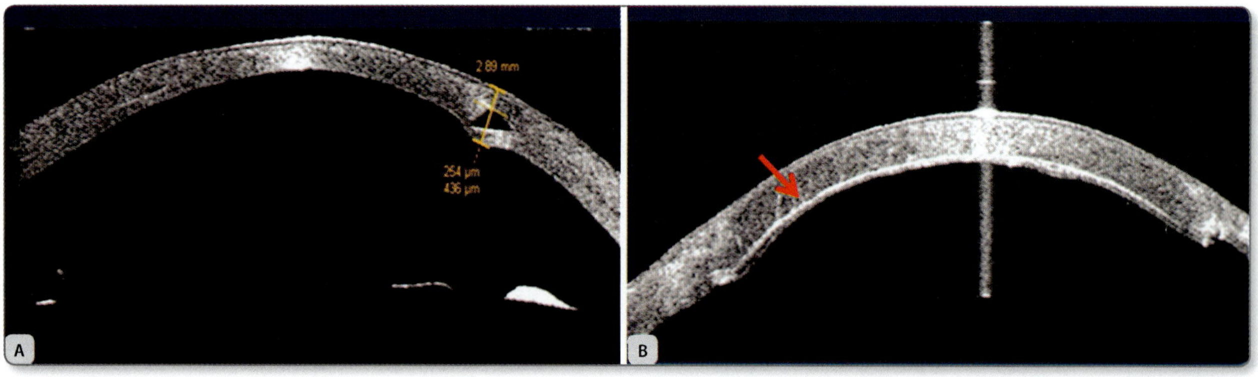

Figs 9.17A and B: Case 1: (A) Preoperative optical coherence tomography (OCT) image showing the corneal thinning and the cross-section of the intracorneal ring segment before the femtosecond (FS) assisted deep anterior lamellar keratoplasty (DALK) procedure; (B) the same patient 2 weeks after the surgical procedure; the white hyperreflective line pointed with the red arrow corresponds to the interface between the recipient and the donor tissue

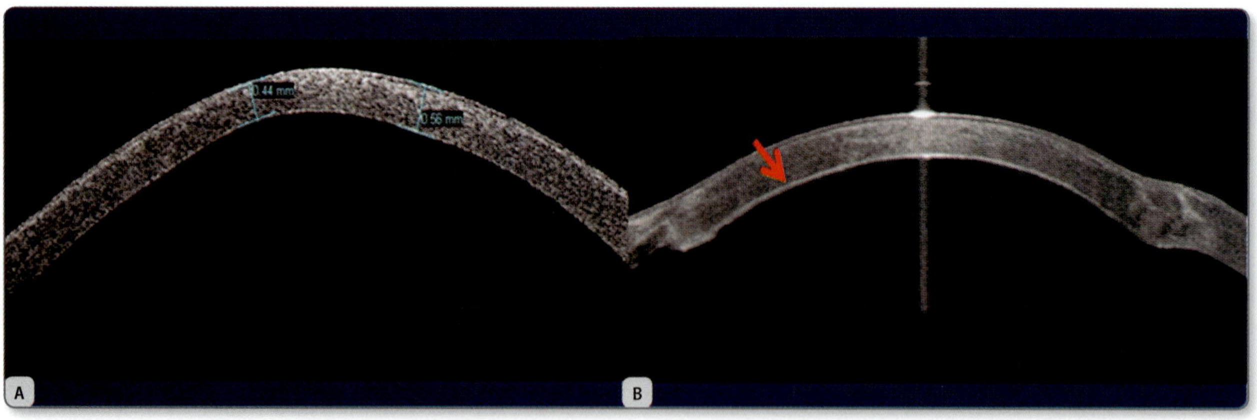

Figs 9.18A and B: Case 2: (A) Preoperative optical coherence tomography (OCT) image showing the corneal thinning of a patient with keratoconus before the femtosecond (FS) assisted deep anterior lamellar keratoplasty (DALK) procedure; (B) the same patient 2 weeks after the surgical procedure; it can be noticed that in this case, the white hyperreflective line pointed with the red arrow is almost imperceptible; this means that in this case, the plane of cleavage during the manual dissection was just above the Descemet's membrane (DM)

Most of the clinical investigations reported as one of the main complication of keratoplasty procedures the high amount of refractive error is mainly related to the induction of irregular astigmatism.[1,12-14] Although there is not a total agreement within the results published in the literature, most investigations found an induction of astigmatism after DALK procedure between 2 diopters and 5 diopters.[13-16] In relation to the spherical equivalent (SE) induced by this technique, most of the published data reported in the literature shows results that goes from a mean of +2 diopters to –5 diopters of SE.[17-19]

Regarding the best corrected visual acuity (BCVA), a mean vision 1 year after the procedure of 20/40 ranging from 20/100 to 20/20 have been reported in most of the scientific data published.[12,15-17, 20-22] Some authors that have studied the effect of the stromal residual bed after DALK procedure have found that there is a correlation between the tissue remaining after baring the DM and the vision that the patient can achieve after the surgery.[20, 22] Those authors have shown that the less the stromal residual tissue is remaining over the DM, the better the outcomes in terms of visual acuity after the procedure.

In terms of graft rejection, endothelial-mediated rejection is unlikely to occur in DALK procedures, as this tissue is not being replaced during the surgery. Nevertheless, epithelial or stromal rejection still can occur, although this type of immune rejection responds well to treatment in comparison with the endothelial rejection. In the study performed by the American Academy of Opthalmology[1] where they retrospectively analyzed the published peer review literature, it was found that around 1% of the cases study presented an episode of immune rejection. All these cases were successfully treated with topical corticosteroid. Neovascularization of the interface is by far the most common factor trigging the immune response against the donor tissue in patients that underwent DALK surgeries.

Another topic of interest when evaluating outcomes after keratoplasty is the endothelial cell population after the surgery. It is a well-known fact that the endothelial cell count presents a major decrease after PK. Some studies report a mean percentage of 74% of endothelial cell lost 10 years after PK. On the other hand, studies that have compared the endothelial cell count between DALK and PK have found a higher cell density in those patients operated of DALK during a follow-up period ranging from 1 year to 5 years.[12, 14, 21, 23, 24] Most of the lost on endothelial cell population after DALK occurs during the first 6 months after the surgery that afterwards shows a stability over a follow-up period of at least 5 years.[7,14] Factors that are related to the loss of endothelial cells after DALK are inherent to the surgical procedure like DM perforation, postoperative pseudoanterior chamber formation, anterior chamber gas injections and air pupillary block. The benefit of long-term endothelial cell survival is clear. Most of the patients that undergo DALK are young patients and avoiding the need of a penetrating procedure will offer them more possibilities of graft survival through their lifetime.

In the recent years, introduction of FS laser in ophthalmology have enhanced the way in which keratoplasty procedures are performed. Although there are still no long follow-up reports, the published data found in the literature shows better outcomes when performing FS assisted keratoplasty procedure in comparison with the manual techniques. A recent study carried out by Gaster et al. reports a better outcomes in terms of visual acuity and topographic astigmatism when comparing the results of patients operated with a FS assisted technique over a mechanical trepanation.[25] In another study where the authors analyzed the variation of IOP and the endothelial cell density after manual or FS assisted keratoplasty, they found that the FS assisted procedure was safer in terms of less variation of the IOP and less endothelial cell damage during the procedure.[26]

In general, the scientific data published in the literature shows that there is no significant difference when comparing the refractive and visual outcomes between DALK and PK procedures. However, the major advantage that DALK procedures provides is related to the low rate of rejection and the benefits related to preserving the endothelial cell for a long period of time in comparison with full LK. On the other hand, with the recent introduction of FS technology to assess keratoplasty procedures, the published data reported the advantage of this technique over the manual dissection in terms of the outcomes related to the visual and corneal astigmatism outcomes.

SUMMARY

Cornea transplant surgery had has a slow development in comparison to other ophthalmological procedures. One of the most important improvements in the last decade in corneal transplant has been the introduction of FS laser technology. This technology has a great acceptance among corneal surgeons because from the surgical standpoint, it is an intuitive technology, easy to learn and capable of improving the results based on its perfect dissection, giving excellent wound apposition and minimizing the suture tension depending of the pattern chosen. However, this technology is not meant to neglect the skills and training of surgeons, we believe that on the contrary, is a technology where the manual procedure remains the most important piece in the transplant surgery. Femtosecond technology represents in this moment the best choice in order to achieve the following goals:

- Excellent wound apposition
- Biomechanical stable incision
- Minimal suture tension thus less induced astigmatism
- Rapid recovery of the wound and vision
- Less invasive surgical procedure.

Despite of all these advantages that FS laser has added to keratoplasty procedures there are still some improvements that have to be done in order to achieve an adequate technique that offers to the patients the best results in terms of functionality and refractive outcomes.

REFERENCES

1. Reinhart WJ, Musch DC, Jacobs DS, et al. Deep anterior lamellar keratoplasty as an alternative to penetrating keratoplasty a report by the American Academy of Ophthalmology. Ophthalmol. 2011;118(1):209-18.
2. DeVoe AG. Ramon Castroviejo. Trans Am Ophthalmol Soc. 1987;85:6-8.
3. Blackmon S, Semchyshyn T, Kim T. Penetrating and lamellar keratoplasty. In: Duane TD, Tasman W, Jaeger EA (Eds). Duane's Clinical Ophthalmology, revised edition. JB Lippincott; 1994.
4. Jhanji V, Sharma N, Vajpayee RB (Eds). Evolution of deep anterior lamellar transplantation. Deep Anterior Lamellar Keratoplasty: Different Strokes, 1st edition. New Delhi: Jaypee Brothers Medical Publishers (P) Ltd; 2012. pp. 3-6.
5. Gasset AR. Lamellar keratoplasty in the treatment of keratoconus: conectomy. Ophthalmic Surg. 1979;10(2):26-33.
6. Sugita J, Kondo J. Deep lamellar keratoplasty with complete removal of pathological stroma for vision improvement. Br J Ophthalmol. 1997;81(3):184-8.
7. van Dooren BT, Mulder PG, Nieuwendaal CP, et al. Endothelial cell density after deep anterior lamellar keratoplasty (Melles technique). Am J Ophthalmol. 2004;137(3):397-400.
8. Anwar M, Teichmann KD. Big-bubble technique to bare Descemet's membrane in anterior lamellar keratoplasty. J Cataract Refract Surg. 2002;28(3):398-403.
9. Farid M, Steinert RF. Deep anterior lamellar keratoplasty performed with the femtosecond laser zig-zag incision for the treatment of stromal corneal pathology and ectatic disease. J Cataract Refract Surg. 2009;35(5):809-13.
10. Slade SG. Applications for the femtosecond laser in corneal surgery. Curr Opin Ophthalmol. 2007;18(4):338-41.
11. Lahners WJ, Culbertson W, Rabinowitz Y, Azar D, Stahl J. (Eds). Femtosecond Laser in Corneal and Refractive Surgery. Online Interactive Ophthalmology Textbook. San Francisco, CA: American Academy of Ophthalmology. 2007.
12. Panda A, Bageshwar LM, Ray M, et al. Deep lamellar keratoplasty versus penetrating keratoplasty for corneal lesions. Cornea. 1999;18(2):172-5.
13. Trimarchi F, Poppi E, Klersy C, et al. Deep lamellar keratoplasty. Ophthalmologica. 2001;215(6):389-93.
14. Krumeich JH, Knülle A, Krumeich BM. Deep anterior lamellar (DALK) vs. penetrating keratoplasty (PKP): a clinical and statistical analysis. Klin Monbl Augenheilkd. 2008;225(7):637-48.
15. Fogla R, Padmanabhan P. Results of deep lamellar keratoplasty using the big-bubble technique in patients with keratoconus. Am J Ophthalmol. 2006;141(2):254-9.
16. Al-Torbak AA, Al-Motowa S, Al-Assiri A, et al. Deep anterior lamellar keratoplasty for keratoconus. Cornea. 2006;25(4):408-12.
17. Shimmura S, Shimazaki J, Omoto M, et al. Deep lamellar keratoplasty (DLKP) in keratoconus patients using viscoadaptive viscoelastics. Cornea. 2005;24(2):178-81.
18. Noble BA, Agrawal A, Collins C, et al. Deep anterior lamellar keratoplasty (DALK): visual outcome and complications for a heterogeneous group of corneal pathologies. Cornea. 2007;26(1):59-64.
19. Villarrubia A, Pérez-Santonja JJ, Palacin E, et al. Deep anterior lamellar keratoplasty in post-laser in situ keratomileusis keratectasia. J Cataract Refract Surg. 2007;33(5):773-8.
20. Ardjomand N, Hau S, McAlister JC, et al. Quality of vision and graft thickness in deep anterior lamellar and penetrating corneal allografts. Am J Ophthalmol. 2007;143(2):228-35.
21. Bahar I, Kaiserman I, Srinivasan S, et al. Comparison of three different techniques of corneal transplantation for keratoconus. Am J Ophthalmol. 2008;146(6):905-12.e1.
22. Alió JL. Visual improvement after late debridement of residual stroma after anterior lamellar keratoplasty. Cornea. 2008;27(8):871-3.
23. Ing JJ, Ing HH, Nelson LR, et al. Ten-year postoperative results of penetrating keratoplasty. Ophthalmol. 1998;105(10):1855-65.
24. Shimazaki J, Shimmura S, Ishioka M, et al. Randomized clinical trial of deep lamellar keratoplasty vs penetrating keratoplasty. Am J Ophthalmol. 2002;134(2):159-65.
25. Gaster RN, Dumitrascu O, Rabinowitz YS. Penetrating keratoplasty using femtosecond laser-enabled keratoplasty with zig-zag incisions versus a mechanical trephine in patients with keratoconus. Br J Ophthalmol. 2012;96(9):1195-9.
26. Angunawela RI, Riau A, Chaurasia SS, et al. Manual suction versus femtosecond laser trephination for penetrating keratoplasty: intraocular pressure, endothelial cell damage, incision geometry, and wound healing responses. Invest Ophthalmol Vis Sci. 2012;53(6):2571-9.

Chapter

10

Femtosecond Laser-Assisted Penetrating Keratoplasty (FLAPK) with WaveLight FS-200 Technology (Use of the Different Technologies, Surgical Practical Pearls, Outcomes)

Georg Gerten

CHAPTER OUTLINE

- Advantages of FLAPK with the WaveLight FS-200 technology
- Published outcomes
- Post-keratoplasty: Astigmatism is still an issue. The suturing technique
- Other treatment options
- Pattern selections and election for FLAPK
- Reducing potential complications
- Standard procedure: Practical tips

INTRODUCTION

It has been more than 8 years since the concept of using the femtosecond (fs) laser in penetrating keratoplasty (PKP) was first discussed and published. Since that time, the femtosecond laser-assisted penetrating keratoplasty (FLAPK, femto-PKP or fs-PKP) has been widely adopted, while the number of fs lasers commercially available has grown to six.[1-5]

When the procedure was introduced, it was heralded as the first breakthrough in corneal surgery in more than 40 years and the results quickly demonstrated improved visual results, quicker healing and lower complication rates. In fact, it is convincing, how perfect the shape of graft and host fit together if both are cut with the same fs laser profile (Figs 10.1A to C).

The perfect fit of graft/host wound bed may have an impact on the optical quality of the transplanted eye (Figs 10.2A to C). It has been speculated that fs laser-cuts lead to lower amounts of regular astigmatism and higher order aberrations ("irregular astigmatism") than manual trephination. But post-keratoplasty optical performance depends on many variable factors in addition to trephination, including underlying corneal disease, suture technique, wound healing, immunology, donor cornea, etc. Large, ongoing data collection and strict study protocols are required to statistically verify an advantage of fs-cuts over manual trephination regarding post-keratoplasty regular astigmatism and higher order aberrations (Figs 10.2B and C).

In 2011, Chamberlin et al. reported on the 2-year follow-up comparing outcomes in patients who underwent an fs-PKP versus conventional PKP and found that the fs eyes showed a significant improvement in astigmatism up to the 6-month postoperative mark. These eyes also underwent earlier suture removal, although there was not a significant difference in best spectacle-corrected visual acuity (BSCVA) at any time point.[6] A study published by Farid et al. also compared results between conventional PKP and fs-PKP showed similar results in terms of astigmatism, but reported that the fs-PKP eyes recovered BSCVA more quickly.[7]

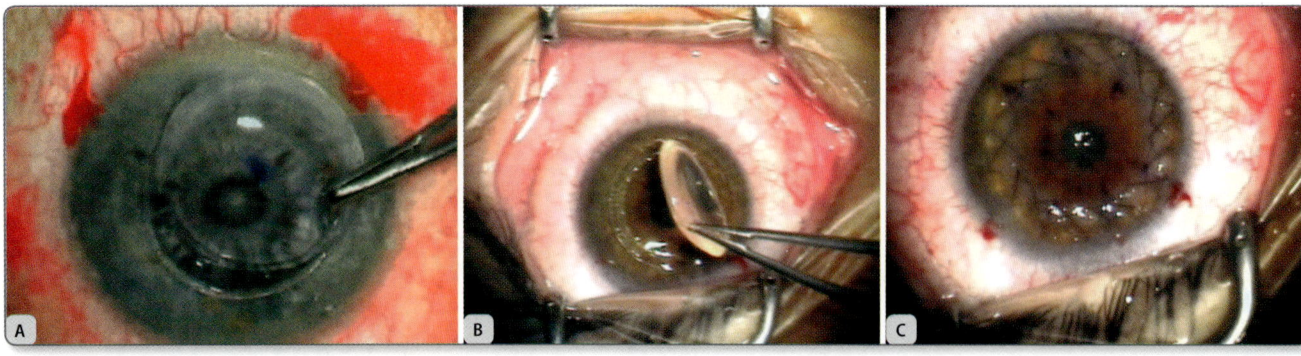

Figs 10.1A to C: Femtosecond laser profiles intraoperative. (A) Top hat step: The transplant is inserted into the recipient bed, "top hat step" at the transplant edge is visible, with a perfect fit; (B) Mushroom step: The transplant is inserted into the recipient bed, "mushroom step" with a perfect fit; (C) Final step of the femtosecond laser-assisted perforating keratoplasty (fs-PKP): The Hoffmann suture is completed, optimal wound compression, stable anterior chamber

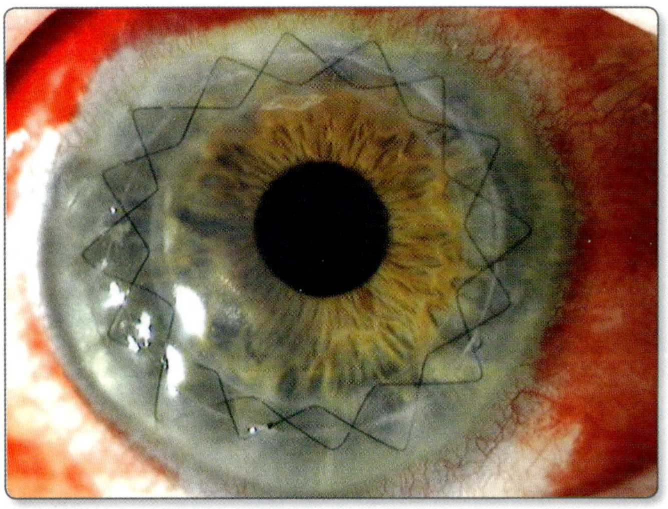

Fig. 10.2A: A 61-year-old female patient; 3 days post-femtosecond laser-assisted perforating keratoplasty (fs-PKP). Modified mushroom (8.0 mm epithelial diameter and 6.5 mm endothelial diameter), epithelium closed, transplant clear and well centered

POST-KERATOPLASTY ASTIGMATISM IS STILL AN ISSUE

In fact, post-fs keratoplasty astigmatism is unfinished business. The fs laser with its planar interface surface displaces the curved corneal tissue. This is not a problem in shallow surface parallel cuts, such as creating flaps on normal-shaped corneas. But in steep keratoconic cornea and with deeper fs-cuts, unpredictable tissue displacement through pressure from a plane interface surface becomes relevant. This is one reason why curved or liquid interfaces are currently under development.[8]

Severe significant astigmatism remains an issue after keratoplasty, even those performed with an fs laser, but there are good options to correct it regardless of the technique (laser or conventional). For instance, if a cataract extraction is necessary, corneal astigmatism can be compensated with a toric intraocular lens (IOL) (in pseudophakia with a toric, add on IOL) (Figs 10.3A to C).[9,10]

Other options are laser treatments directly on the cornea.[11] Beside ablation methods [photorefractive keratectomy (PRK), laser-assisted in-situ keratomileusis (LASIK), laser-assisted sub-epithelial keratectomy (LASEK)], incisional procedures like femtolaser arcuate incisions are suitable to treat transplant astigmatism in PKP.[12,13] The femtolaser arcuate cuts should be executed in the transplant, adjacent to the graft/host interface in the steep meridian. With these fs-cuts, up to ~ 8 diopter of astigmatism can be corrected, depending on depth, length and optical zone of the arcuate incisions. These parameters for the arcuate incisions are much more standardized and controlled with the laser as compared to arcuate incisions created with a diamond knife. Still, the refractive effect is difficult to predict precisely; a drawback due to variable anatomy of the individual cornea/transplant. The author uses the IntraLase® fs laser to execute arcuate incisions in order to reduce larger amounts of astigmatism, well aware that a residual astigmatism may persist, which might be in the range of spectacle correction (Figs 10.4A to C).

As mentioned in Chapter 5, the WaveLight® FS-200 fs laser is capable of performing PKP using a top-hat, mushroom or zig-zag configuration. With this laser system, the entry data are entered for the diameter of anterior cut (at the corneal surface) and the posterior cut (at the maximum depth of the cut), the depth of both cuts and then the angle of the cuts. The laser software calculates the lamellar part as a "connection" of the posterior and anterior cut, so its width cannot be entered manually. Table 10.1 and Figure 10.5 provide details about the geometry and laser settings required for the WaveLight® FS-200 laser that the author has adopted at his center. The laser is even able to cut through

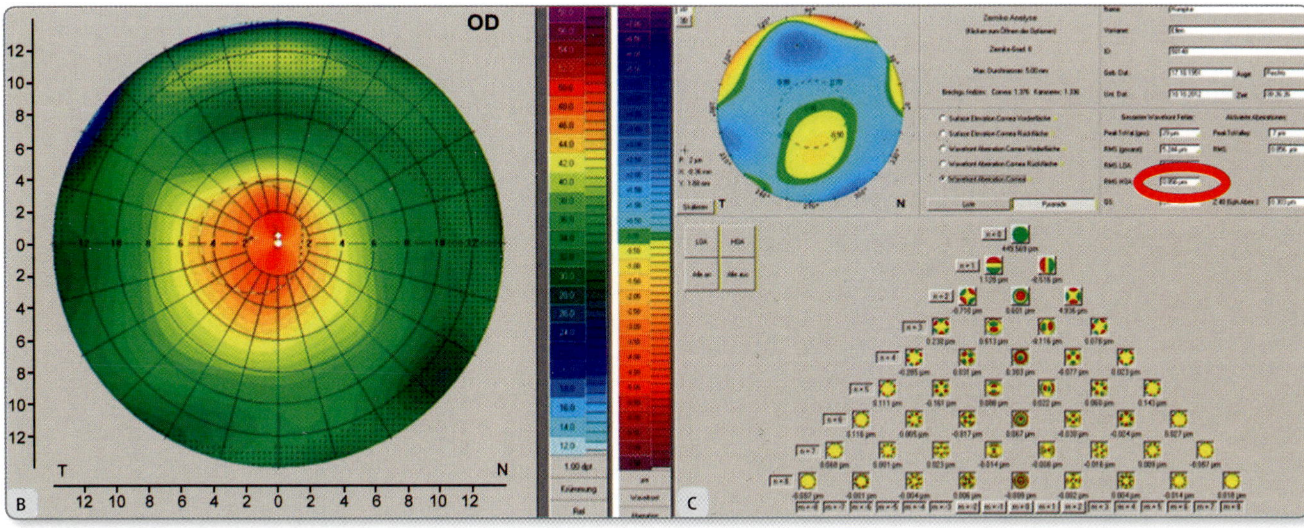

Figs 10.2B and C: Corneal evaluation of the same eye (61-year-old female patient). After suture removal, 1 year post femtosecond keratoplasty based on Scheimpflug photography (*Source*: Pentacam®, Oculus Ltd. Germany). (B) Topography: Transplant provides a smooth and large optical zone overlapping the pupil, astigmatism ~ 2 diopter, grid centered on the corneal apex, pupil margin indicated by dotted line; (C) Zernike decomposition: Mushroom transplant showing low amount of higher order aberrations (~ 0.8 µm, red circle) enabling a spectacle-corrected visual acuity of 1.0p

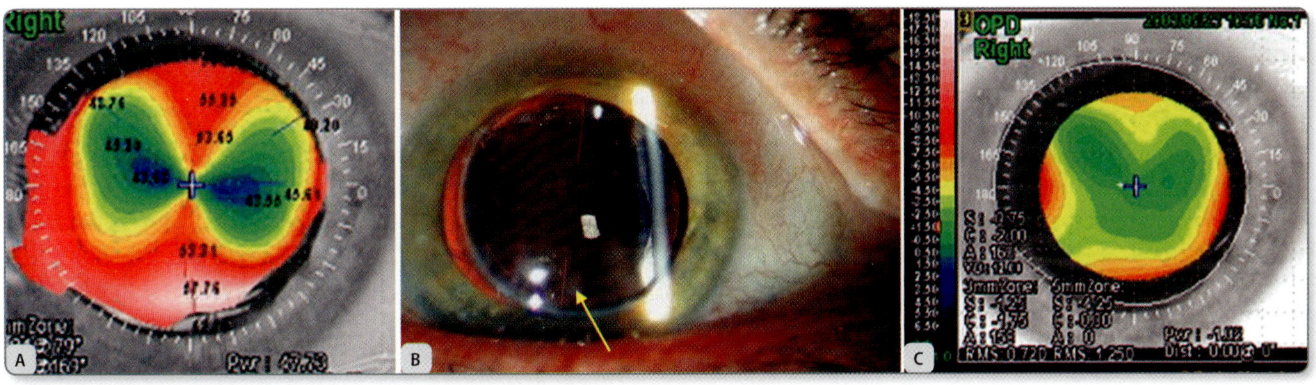

Figs 10.3A to C: Toric intraocular lens (IOL)/artisan IOL to correct regular astigmatism after conventional keratoplasty. (A) Topography showing ~ 7 diopter (central regular part) of post-penetrating keratoplasty (PKP) astigmatism; (B) Toric IOL aligned with the steep meridian of corneal astigmatism in 85° (yellow arrow); (C) Refraction map of the complete optics of the eye (Source: Nidek® OPD). Toric IOL and cornea result in minimal residual astigmatism. Best spectacle corrected visual acuity (BSCVA): - 0.25 – 0.75/152 = 1.0p

light to mid-dense scars, as long as the scar tissue is not vascularized (Figs 10.6A and B).

In corneas with neovascularization, the author treats the pathological vessels in a separate operation before the transplantation. This is done by using a combination of thermal and pharmaceutical treatments: a coagulation of the neovascularization (with an argon laser, electric cautery or a conductive keratoplasty device) together with the sub-Tenon's application of bevacizumab. Four to six weeks after a single or repeated treatment, the neovascularization is reduced sufficiently to enable surgery to proceed with the fs laser in approximately 50% of all eyes. The remaining eyes required surgery using a conventional mechanical approach.

REDUCING POTENTIAL COMPLICATIONS

Although the use of the fs laser for therapeutic corneal procedures has improved the safety and efficacy of the procedure, immunology is still a concern. If corneal pathology is limited to a paracentral area, an fs-autologous rotational keratoplasty can be considered (Figs 10.7A and B).[14]

However, there remain some intraoperative risks with the fs laser approach to PKP. As the recipient's eye is completely destabilized after the fs-cut of the central cornea, the lenticle is loose, which could result in the contents of the eye protruding through the opening. This is

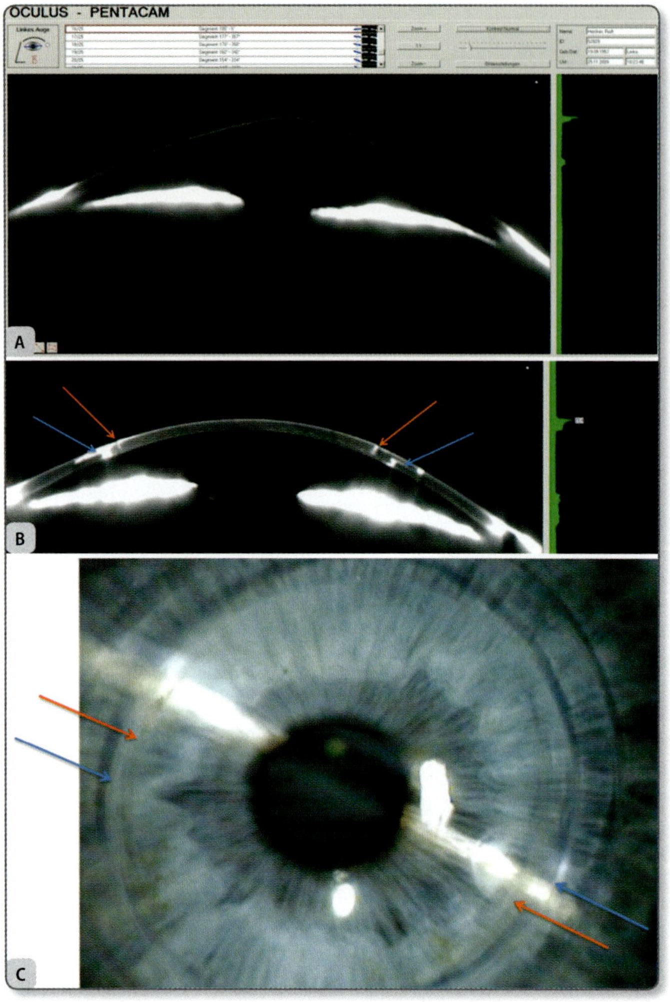

Figs 10.4A to C: (A) A Scheimpflug image of a keratoconus grade III cornea pre-femtosecond laser-assisted penetrating keratoplasty (fs-PKP); (B) A Scheimpflug image of the same cornea post-fs PKP (mushroom profile) and post arcuate incisions (red arrows, femtolaser arcuate incisions; blue arrows, graft/host interface); (C) Slit-lamp picture of same cornea showing fs-arcuate incisions in the steep meridian (6-mm zone, 80° arc length). The incisions reduced the graft astigmatism by 6 diopter (red arrows, femtolaser arcuate incisions; blue arrows, inner graft/host interface)

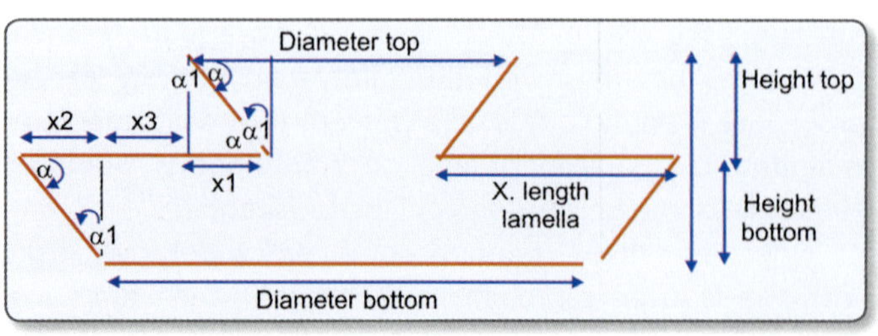

Fig. 10.5: Possible geometry for a modified top-hat corneal graft with the WaveLight® FS-200 laser

Table 10.1: Geometry and laser settings required for the WaveLight® FS-200 laser

	Recipient	*Donor*	*Donor*	*Donor*
		epithlium on	epithelium off	epi off/D1 fit
Pachy Patient/ Donor [μm]	550	800	800	
Other +/-[μm]	100	100	50	
Thickness [mm]	450	900	850	850
Diamter Top [mm]	8.0	8.0	8.0	7.8
Diameter Bottom [mm]	6.2	4.6	4.8	4.8
Height Top [μm]	250	250	200	200
Height Bottom [μm]	200	650	650	650
Angle to Femto α	30	30	30	30
Angle Top Stroma α1	60	60	60	60
Angle Bottom Stroma α1	60	60	60	60
Angle Bottom Femto α	30	30	30	30
				86.60
X1 [μm]	433.01	433.01	346.41	346.41
X2 [μm]	346.41	1125.83	1125.83	1125.83
X3 [μm]	-900.00	-1679.42	-1592.82	-1592.82
x: length lamella [μm]	-120.58	-120.58	-120.58	-120.58
mismatch [μm]		20.6	7.2	7.2

a major drawback while the patient is moved between the laser and the surgical microscope to finish the operation, particularly if the surgical rooms are on different levels or even buildings.

To overcome these risks, the author's team has developed what they call the "3 bridges" technique, which utilizes a disposable mask to provide an additional safety feature while moving the patient. This is accomplished by leaving well-defined tissue bridges to prevent the trephined corneal part from blowing out. The approach leaves a thin layer of corneal tissue at three quadrants, providing an additional margin of safety while the patient is transferred to the operating microscope (Figs 10.8A and B).

STANDARD PROCEDURE

The author's team has performed fs-laser assisted keratoplasties since 2004 with different laser systems,

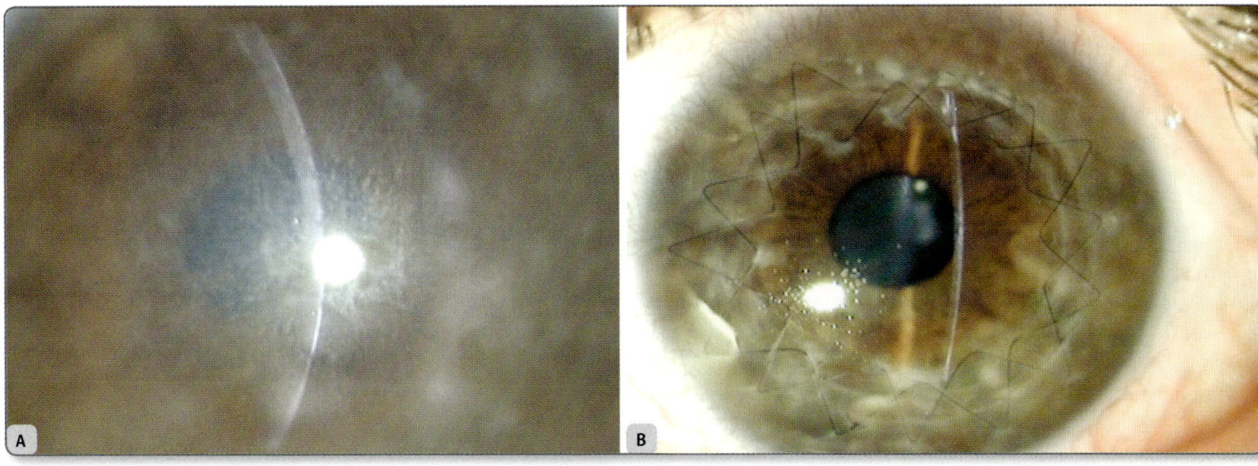

Figs 10.6A and B: (A) A corneal opacification in a 28-year-old male patient with macular dystrophy; (B) The same patient 1.2 years after femtosecond laser-assisted penetrating keratoplasty (fs-PKP). Intraoperatively, energy was set to the maximum (2.4 µJ) and the fs laser was able to create a complete cut through the opaque corneal tissue

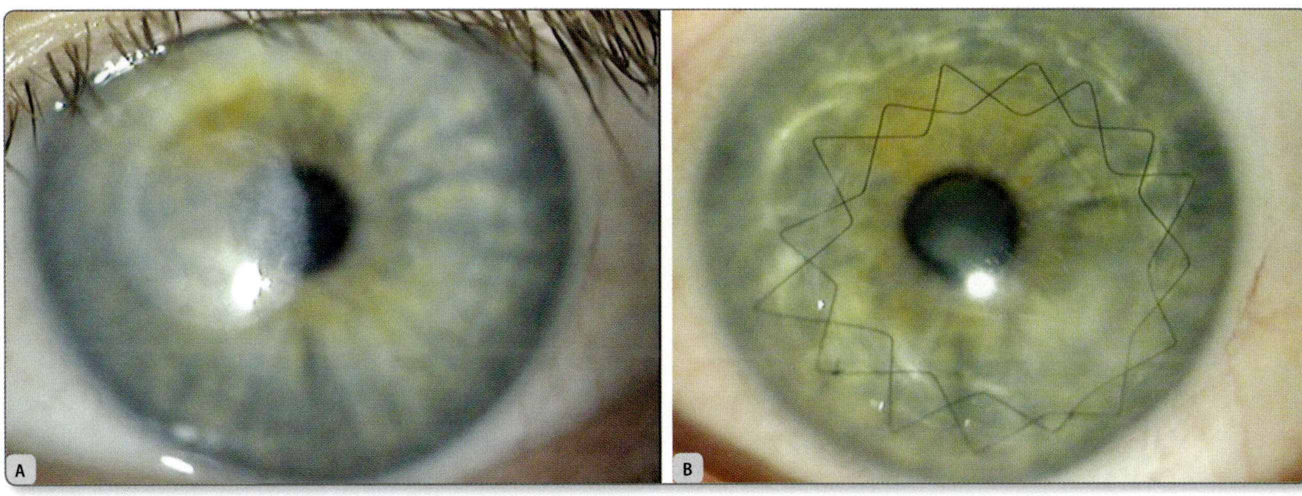

Figs 10.7A and B: Femtosecond-autologous rotational keratoplasty. (A) A corneal scar (infection after corneal foreign body) in a 63-year-old male patient; (B) The same patient 6 weeks after autologous femtosecond laser-assisted penetrating keratoplasty (fs-PKP). By rotating the central cornea, the scarred nasal inferior zones are replaced by the temporal and superior quadrants

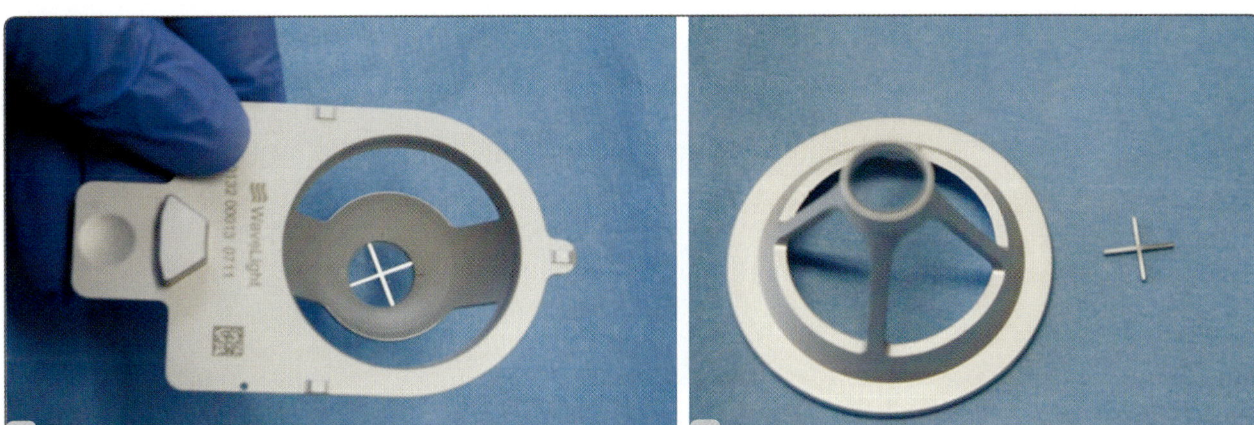

Figs 10.8A and B: These newly developed disposable masks (*Source*: Geuder® AG, Heidelberg, Germany) enables the creation of four "tissue bridges" (previous mask had three bridges) that provide corneal stability as the patient is moved

performing both full thickness keratoplasties, as well as lamellar procedures. The fs-PKP group contains a subgroup with ~ 50 patients that were treated with a modified mushroom laser pattern. The modified mushroom configuration is one of the typical femtosecond-laser assisted keratoplasty procedures that the author's team performs with the FS-200 now. Here, they discussed their initial results from the first five patients, scheduled for fs-PKP due to progressive keratoconus, using the "3 bridges" technique with the custom-made device to shield a part of the laser beam (Figs 10.9A to R).

The procedures were performed with the IntraLase™ FS-60 or the WaveLight® FS-200 fs laser. The disposable device consists of three (or four) arms with a width of 1 mm. This device is placed on top of the contact glass of the fs laser in order to prevent photodisruption just beneath the arms of the mask, thereby preventing any tissue separation in this specified narrow region. In order to limit the photodisruption to the upper part of the zig-zag/mushroom pattern in the cornea, laser emission was stopped at a depth ~ 100–130 µm

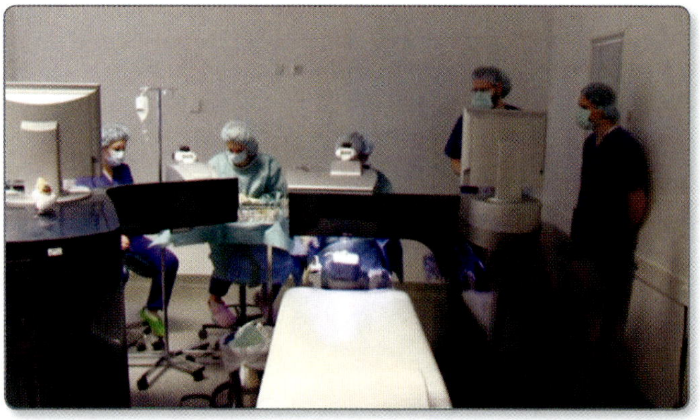

Fig. 10.9A: Transplant laser trephination is prepared

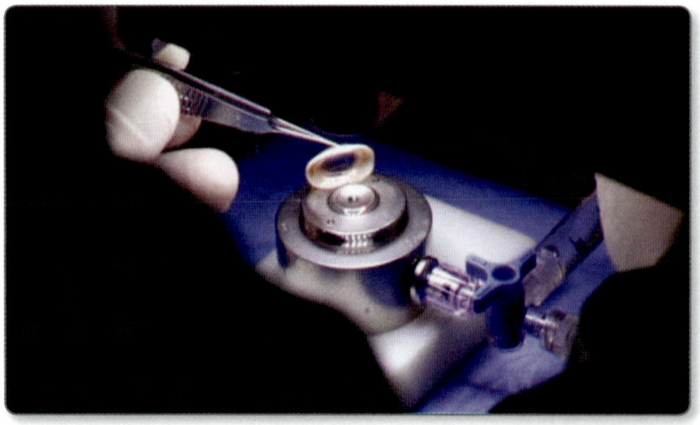

Fig. 10.9B: The transplant is mounted on a modified artificial anterior chamber
Source: GTS® System, Polytech® Ophthalomologie, Rossdorf, Germany

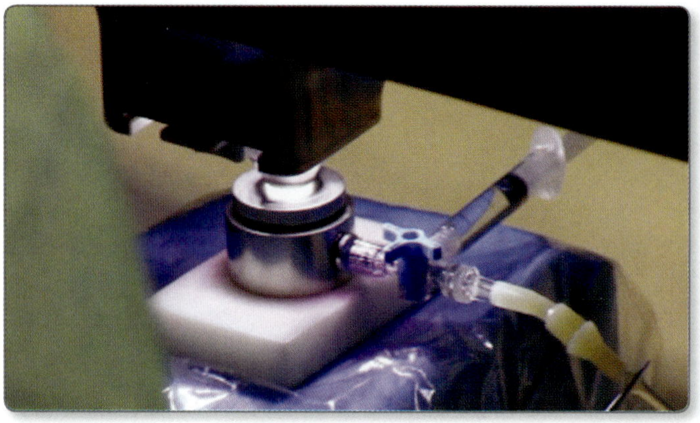

Fig. 10.9C: The WaveLight® FS-200 fs laser interface is connected to the transplant surface

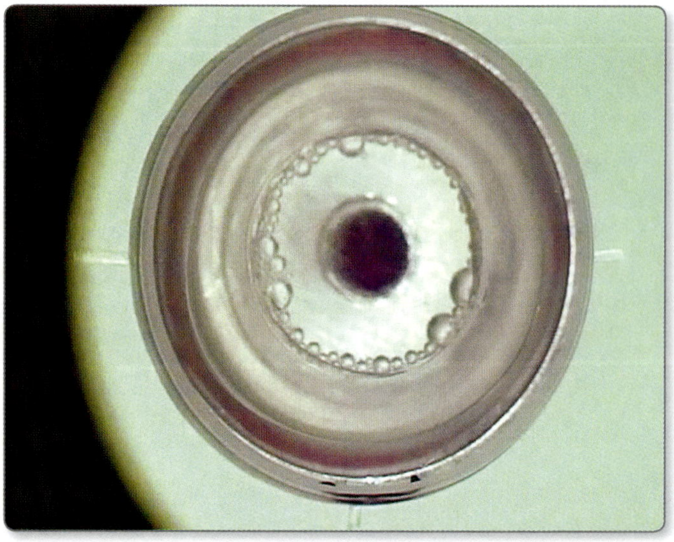

Fig. 10.9D: The femtosecond (fs)-cut is performed in the transplant

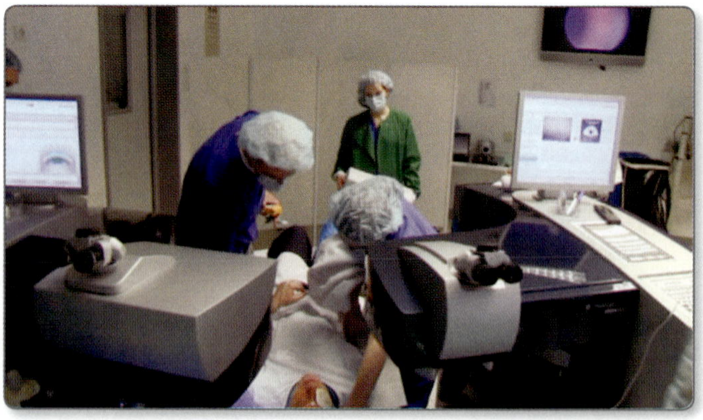

Fig. 10.9E: The patient is placed under the laser

before epithelial breakthrough, which corresponds to ~ 80% of the overall procedure (depending on the laser pattern). Then the mask was introduced into the interface and the

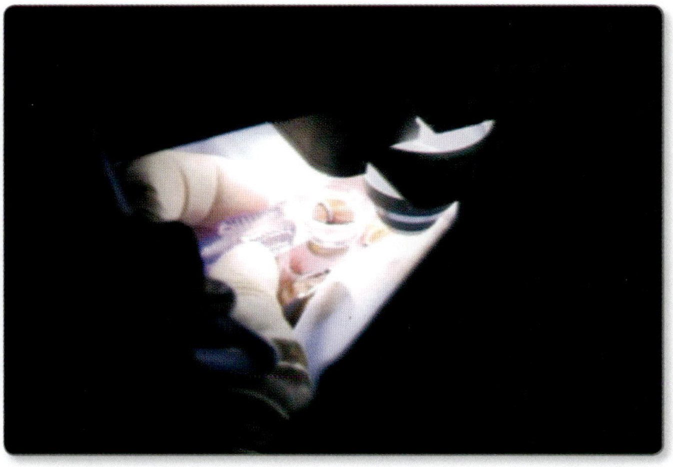

Fig. 10.9F: The suction ring is placed on the patient's eye

rest of the laser pattern was executed. This limits the depth of the bridged tissue (side cuts) to ~ 130 µm, which means that it does not interfere with non-surface-perpendicular deeper parts of the laser pattern. This guarantees that the opening of the bridges can be done easily under the microscope later on without compromising the transplant edges. No other changes to the setup of the laser are necessary.

Upon completion of the fs laser ablation, the patients were transferred to the operating room as per author's standard procedure. Once the patients were placed under the operating microscope, the surgery was completed as normal with easy dissection of the three points of distinct local stromal bridges. Due to the shielding mask in the laser beam, very distinct corneal bridges of stromal tissue can be achieved, preventing an accidental opening of the cornea

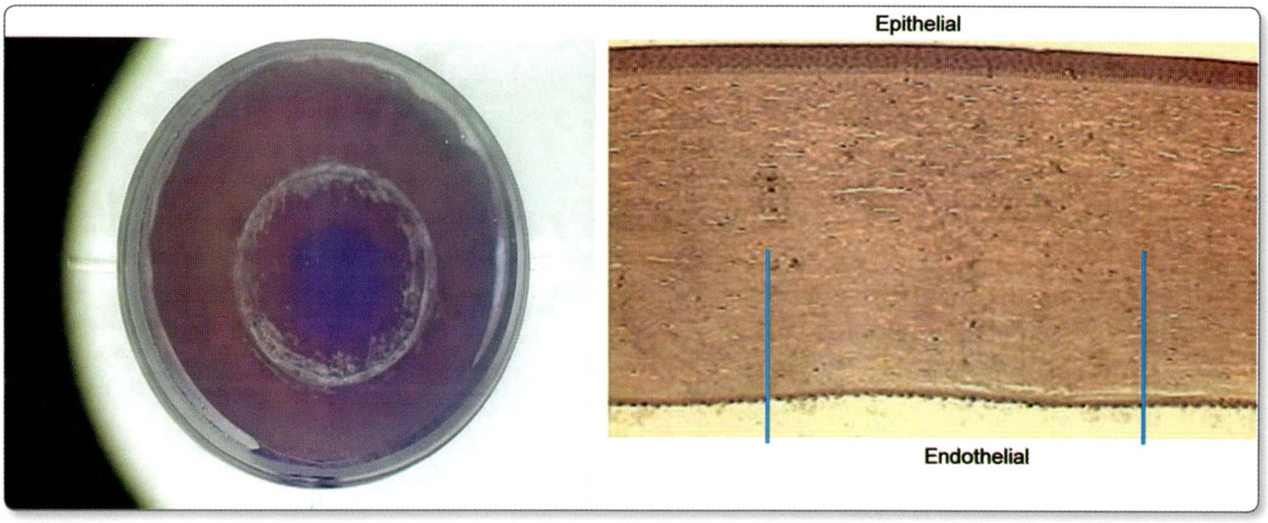

Fig. 10.9G: The femtosecond (fs) laser starts photodisruption in the anterior chamber and is moving upwards into the posterior stroma of the keratoconic eye

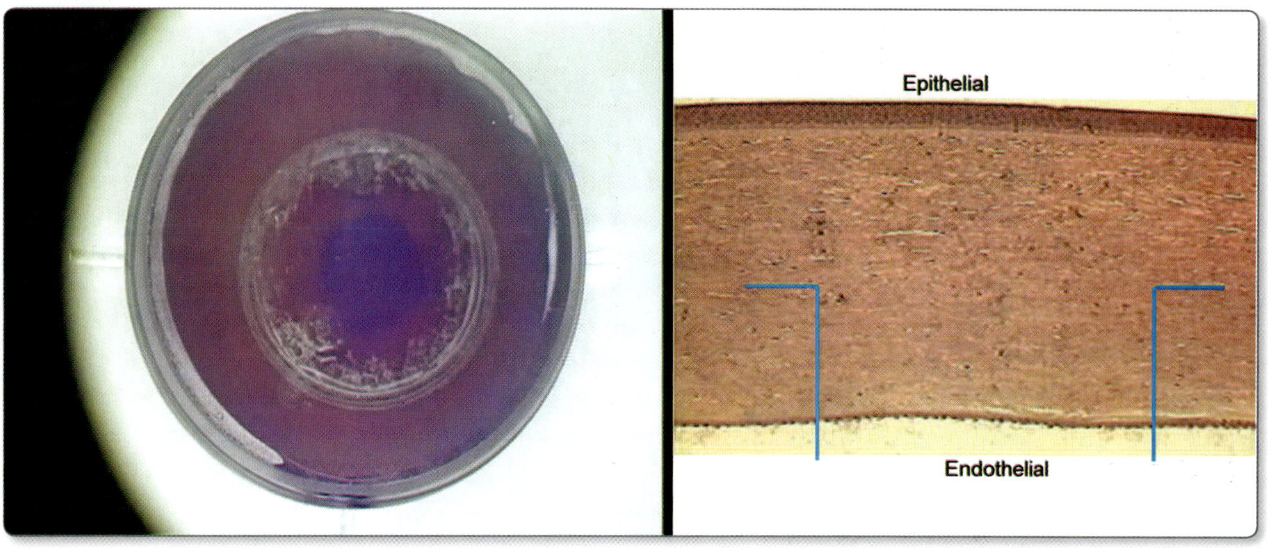

Fig. 10.9H: The femtosecond (fs) laser is executing the surface parallel cut of the mushroom profile step

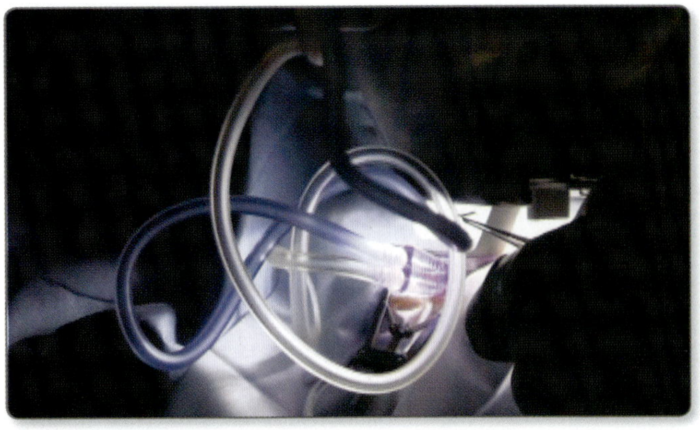

Fig. 10.9I: The femtosecond (fs) laser pattern is ~ 80% complete. The surgeon stops the laser and drops the mask (here a "3 bridges" type mask) into the interface cone

as a result of extraocular/intraocular pressure changes. The eyes showed a stable anterior chamber after fs trephination. Light microscopy histology found that the corneal bridges are located only in the upper part of the cornea with precisely defined edges. The three bridges could be cut easily using a simple steel blade any time during the operation without any impact on cut quality. The remaining steps of the PKP procedure—central corneal replacement and suturing were uneventful. At 1-week postoperative, the corneal graft was well positioned and the anterior chamber was quiet (Figs 10.9A to R).

The "3 bridges" technique for fs-laser-assisted trephination showed improved safety by maintaining a closed anterior chamber. It is even possible to do a phacoemulsification in this closed system. However, to further facilitate the phacoprocedure and IOL implantation, the author's team is currently developing a "4 bridges system". The "4 bridges system" approach is designed to secure the anterior chamber stability, even in difficult cases where increased intraocular manipulation is required. As a result, with this "4 bridges" approach, even triple procedures can be done with safe phacoemulsification and IOL implantation after the fs-laser cuts have been performed on the cornea. As soon as the IOL is placed, the four tissue bridges can be opened to complete the corneal transplantation.

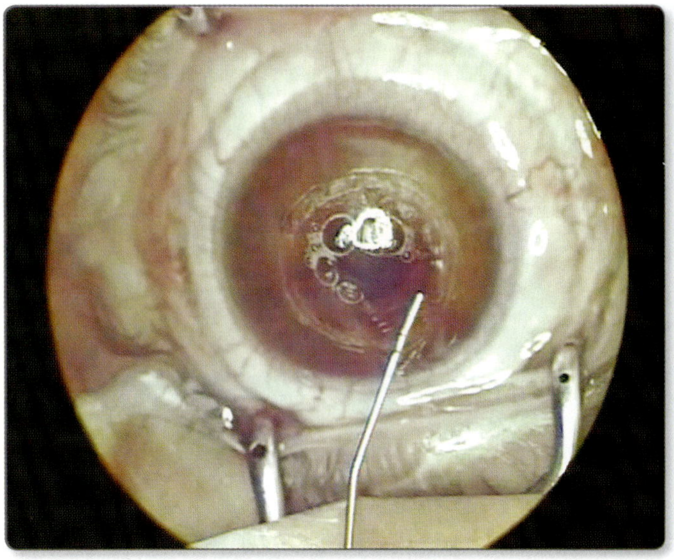

Fig. 10.9K: The femtosecond (fs) laser trephination of the recipient cornea is completed. The bridges secure a stable anterior chamber, which is filled with an ophthalmic viscosurgical device (OVD) of high viscosity

This is now author's preferred method for performing this procedure. Of course the "bridge concept" could be

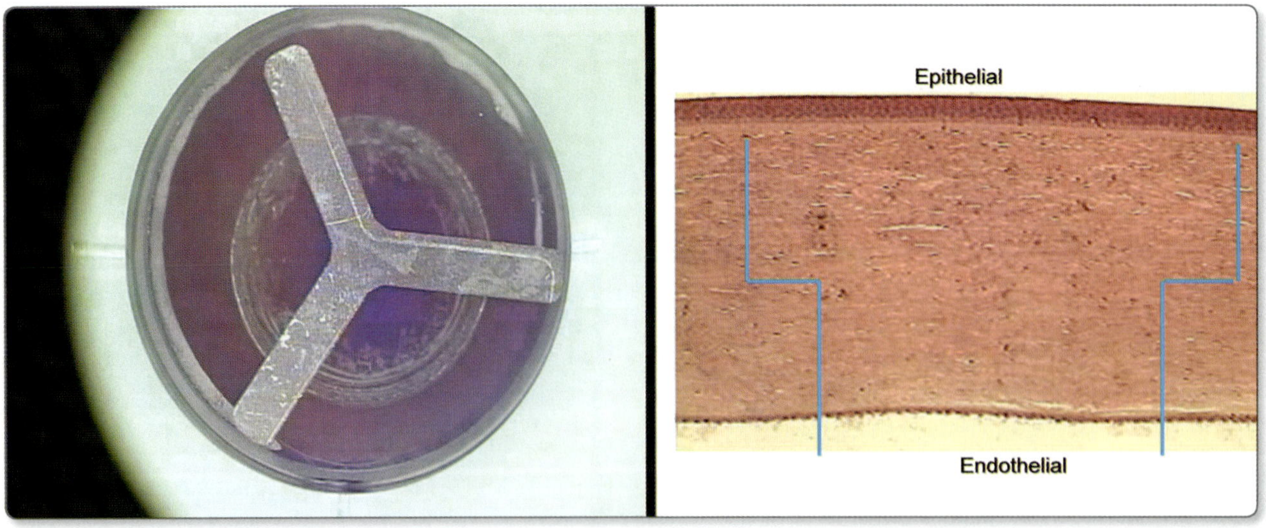

Fig. 10.9J: The mask is inserted into the cone. The surgeon enables the laser again to finish the pattern

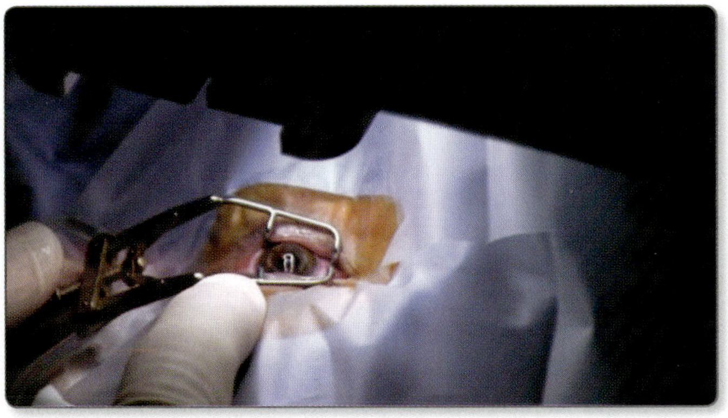

Fig. 10.9L: The lid speculum is removed

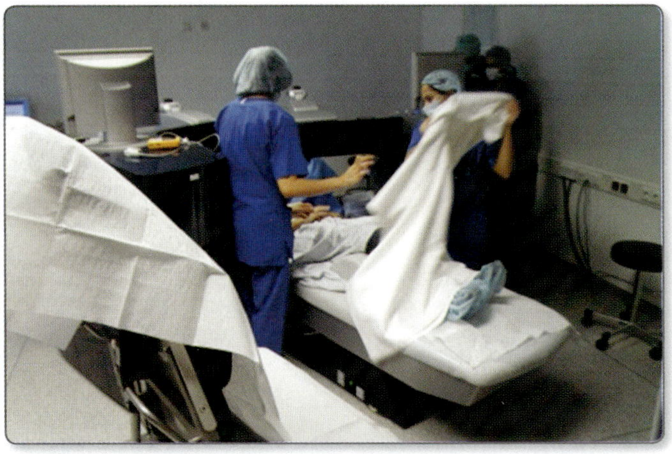

Fig. 10.9M: After femtosecond (fs)-laser trephination, the patient is transferred to an operating room equipped with a microsurgery unit

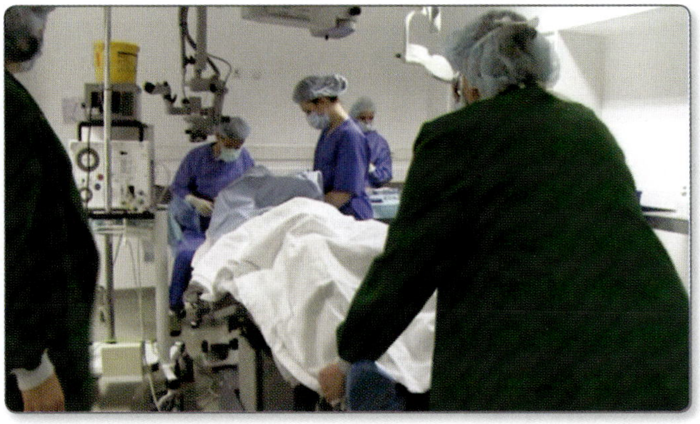

Fig. 10.9N: The patient is positioned under the microscope

achieved by reprogramming the femtolaser pattern for every laser as well. But this is technically demanding, time consuming and binds the human resources of the laser companies' research teams. Furthermore, a new US Food

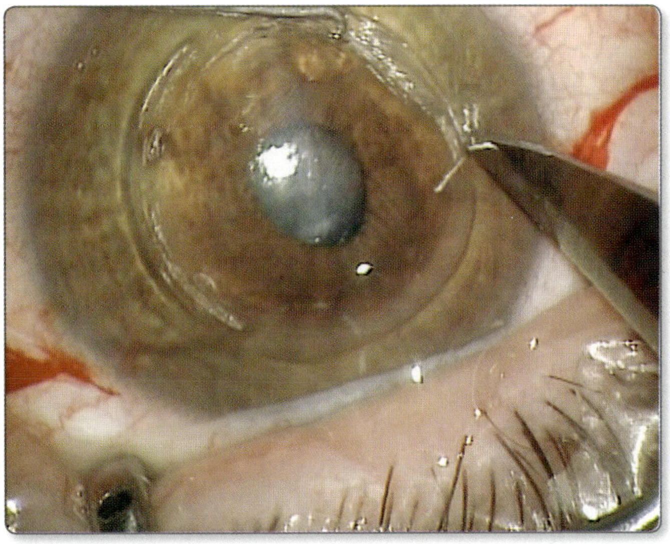

Fig. 10.9O: The tissue bridges are opened and the central keratoconic recipient cornea is easily removed

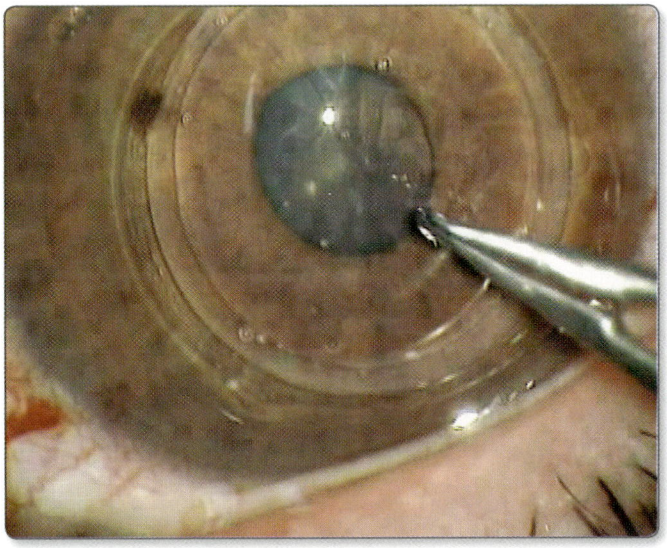

Fig. 10.9P: The transplant fits perfectly

and Drug Administration (FDA) and Conformit Europe (CE, Europe) admission process is required.

SUTURE TECHNIQUE REMAINS IMPORTANT

Due to the angle of the zig-zag or modified mushroom femtolaser profile, the wound surfaces of the donor and recipient have a larger contact zone than with mechanical or solely perpendicular fs-cuts. So femtotransplant fit ideally into the wound architecture of the recipient and

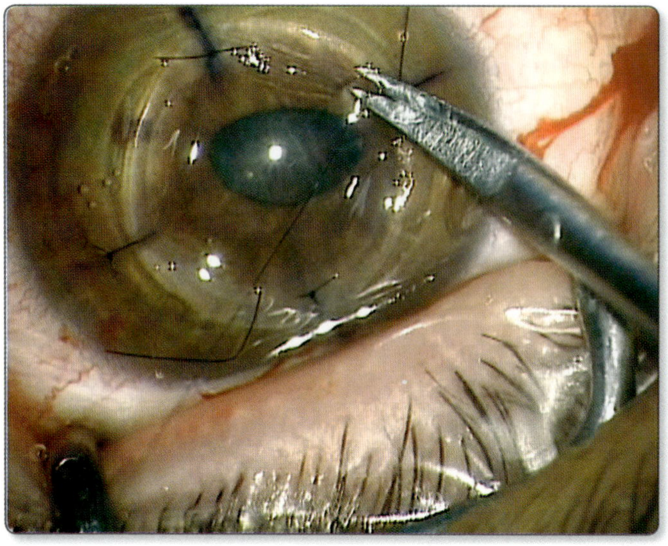

Fig. 10.9Q: The rudiments of the tissue bridges (with four bridges mask only) can be used as landmarks for the four cardinal sutures to place the transplant exactly without tissue stress

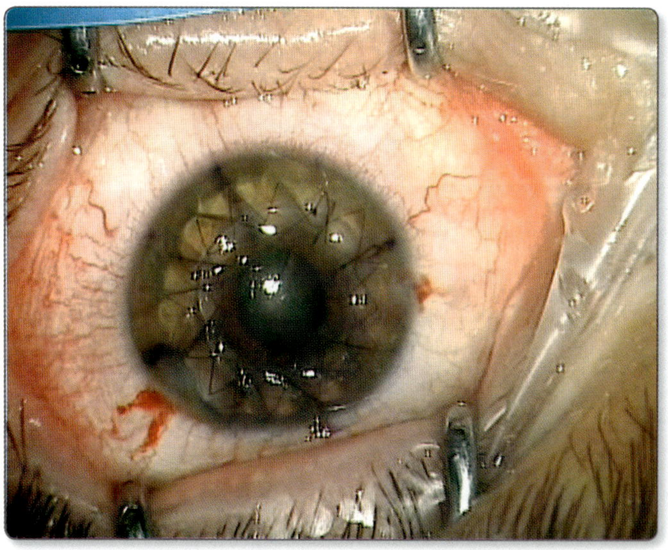

Fig. 10.9R: The final step of the femtosecond laser-assisted penetrating keratoplasty (fs-PKP): the Hoffmann suture is completed, with perfect wound adaption and a stable anterior chamber
Source: Video available from youtube/xhY2paU8EiE or www.youtube.com/user/augenportal1

the transplanted eye is more stable and in principle, should show a rapid healing.[6] Consequently, safe suture removal should be possible earlier in the postoperative recovery. However, another precondition for consistent healing is tight compression between the wound surfaces. If mechanical stability is guaranteed, stable collagen filaments can be established through the wound interface to connect donor and recipient tissue (Figs 10.10B and C). In fact, wound surfaces with sliding movements prevent permanent collagen bridges from developing.

The author's team experienced this phenomenon when they tried to fixate a transplant with eight single sutures only. Since this case, they have changed their suturing technique to the use of a double-running, anti-torque, Hoffmann suture (10:0 Nylon).[15] This approach allows us to achieve stable and rapid wound adoption in all cases (Fig. 10.9R and Figs 10.10A to C). With this method, the sutures can be removed earlier than in mechanical PKPs, on average. Usually between 6 months and 1.5 years post-PKP, depending on the clinical course.

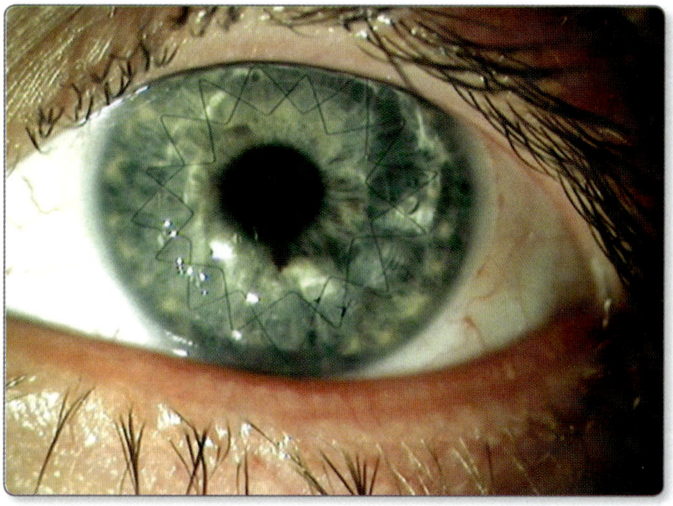

Fig. 10.10A: One month post-fs-keratoplasty with "4 bridges technique" (modified mushroom laser pattern). Well centered and clear transplant (epithelial diameter 7.9 mm) with 0.8 mm overlap zone shows perfect adaption with double running anti-torque Hoffmann suture, visual acuity 0.5p

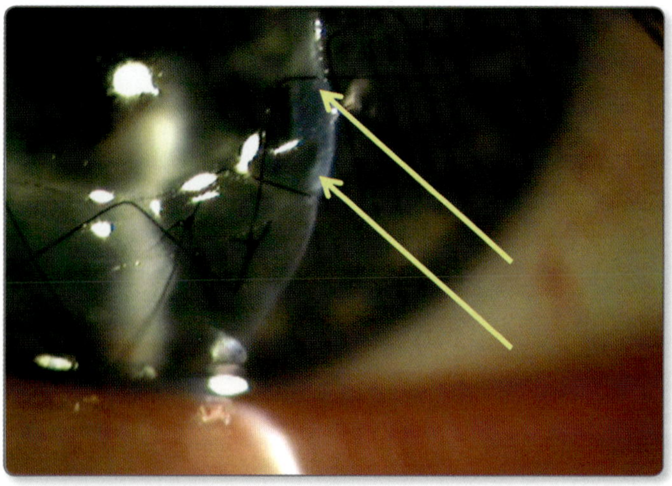

Fig. 10.10B: Slit-lamp photograph 1-month post-femtosecond laser-assisted penetrating keratoplasty (fs-PKP). Transplant (visible back-scattering of light, yellow arrows) and recipient cornea shows well-adapted wound architecture due to modified mushroom laser pattern

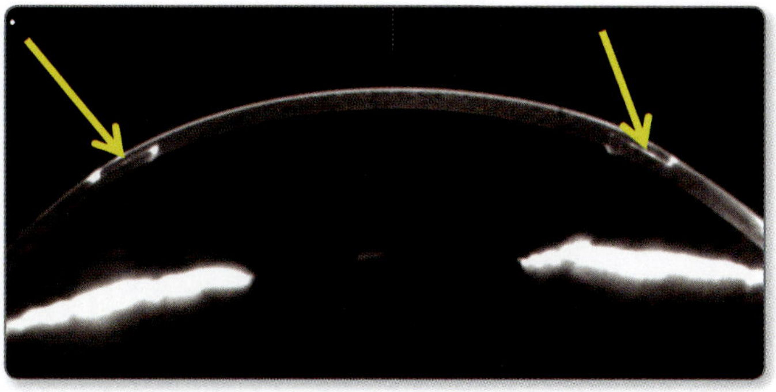

Fig. 10.10C: Scheimpflug image 2-year post femtosecond laser-assisted penetrating keratoplasty (fs-PKP). High interface reflectivity (yellow arrows) indicating healing response

The use of a fs-laser for performing PKP is now author's team standard procedure when patients require a full-thickness procedure. The described procedure is straightforward, wound healing is quicker and patients' recover vision more quickly than what they experienced with the mechanical approach.

REFERENCES

1. Lubatschowski H. Overview of commercially available femtosecond lasers in refractive surgery. J Refract Surg. 2008;24:S102-7.
2. Gerten G. Bevacizumab (Avastin) and argon laser to treat neovascularization in corneal transplant surgery. Cornea. 2008;27:1195-9.
3. Lubatschowski H, The ROWIAK Femtosecond Laser in the CE Mark admission Process, Personal Communication. Rowiak GmbH, October 2012
4. Jonas JB, Vossmerbaeumer U. Femtosecond laser penetrating keratoplasty with conical incisions and positional spikes. J Refract Surg. 2004;20:397.
5. Seitz B, Brünner H, Viestenz A, et al. Inverse mushroom-shaped nonmechanical penetrating keratoplasty using a femtosecond laser. Am J Ophthalmol. 2005;139:941-4.
6. Meltendorf C, Schroeter J, Bug R, et al. Corneal trephination with the femtosecond laser. Cornea. 2006;25:1090-2.
7. Slade SG. Applications for the femtosecond laser in corneal surgery. Curr Opin Ophthalmol. 2007;18:338-41.
8. Tan DT, Mehta JS. Future directions in lamellar corneal transplantation. Cornea. 2007;26:S21-8.
9. Chamberlain WD, Rush SW, Mathers WD, et al. Comparison of femtosecond laser-assisted keratoplasty versus conventional penetrating keratoplasty. Ophthalmol. 2011;118:486-91.
10. Farid M, Steinert RF, Gaster RN, et al. Comparison of penetrating keratoplasty performed with a femtosecond laser zig-zag incision versus conventional blade trephination. Ophthalmol. 2009;116:1638-43.
11. Gerten G, Michels A, Olmes A. Toric intraocular lenses. Clinical results and rotational stability. Ophthalmologe (Germany). 2001;98:715-20.
12. Hodge C, Sutton G, Lawless M, et al. Photorefractive keratectomy with mitomycin-C after corneal transplantation for keratoconus. J Cataract Refract Surg. 2011;37:1884-94.
13. Buzzonetti L, Petrocelli G, Laborante A, et al. Arcuate keratotomy for high postoperative keratoplasty astigmatism performed with the IntraLase femtosecond laser. J Refract Surg. 2009;25:709-14.
14. Consultation section. Cataract surgical problem december consultation #1. J Cataract Refract Surg. 2011;37:2225-30.
15. Hoffmann F. Die Kreuznaht für die perforierende Keratoplastik. Klin Monbl Augenheilkd. 1978;173:696-700.

Chapter

11

Femtosecond Laser-Assisted Endothelial Lamellar Keratoplasty: Optimizing Endothelial Graft Preparation: Laser Setting and Results

Jean-Louis Bourges

CHAPTER OUTLINE

- Cutting profiles for posterior lamellar keratoplasty
  - Single pass and double pass profiles
  - Double layer profile
  - Mixed procedures
  - Preparation from endothelial side
- Laser settings and optimization of the surgical technique
- Clinical outcomes : The actual position of femtosecond assisted posterior lamellar graft for the practical surgeon

INTRODUCTION

Endothelial lamellar keratoplasty (ELK) requires the creation of a posterior stromal button from a donor cornea to selectively replace a damaged endothelium. The endothelial button (or lenticule) can either be prepared with a microkeratome or with a femtosecond laser (FS). Microkeratome lamellar dissection is inexpensive, well-standardized and provides buttons with smoother interfaces compared to FS precutting.[1-3] Smoother stromal interfaces could allow for long-term visual outcomes. Still, ELK could benefit from using the FS blade to create lenticules.[4]

Femtosecond laser endothelial keratoplasty (FLEK) emerged 5 years after the first KLE manual technique was reported by Melles et al.[5-7] The first case was reported by Cheng et al. in 2007.[8] It came from the fact that microkeratomes are restricted for depth adjustments while FS lasers allow for precise customization.[9] Shapes of mechanically prepared buttons also demonstrate poor reproducibility,[10] whereas FSs excel in accuracy, reproducibility and standardization.[11-15] The regularity of the buttons is preserved in case of abortion of the FS procedure whereas the same incident could result in a damaging stromal projection under mechanical preparation.[16] Planar-shaped buttons are obtained easily.[17] Although it is a theoretical concern, the rate of postoperative complications was reported to be similar to mechanical procedures.[18] So far FLEK procedure demonstrates disappointing visual outcomes.[2,11] Although graft's thickness seems to impact not much visual outcomes,[19] the lack of smoothness and regularity at graft's interface is likely to generate aberrations combined with photic disturbances, impairing at least in part patient's vision.[20-25]

We explored various cutting profiles and FS laser settings aiming to optimize FLEK and, in the end, to enhance visual results in patients with this procedure.

CUTTING PROFILES

Single Path Profile

Endothelial buttons are usually created with FS, using successive posterior circular side cuts and a lamellar cut performed from the epithelial side of the donor cornea.

The lamellar cut depth is set according to the intraoperative pachymetry. The FS cone is applied on the epithelial side of the donor cornea, which is mounted before on an artificial anterior chamber. Eventually, the endothelial lenticule is dissected in the operating room (OR) from the endothelial side (Fig. 11.1A).

Double Path Profile

The double path cutting profile is similar to the single path except that the lamellar cut is performed twice within a single session of applanation.

Double Layer Profile

The double layer profile includes an initial debulking to thin the anterior stroma of the donor's cornea. Within a first session of applanation, an anterior lenticule is created and removed (Fig. 11.1B), and the residual bed thickness (RBT) is evaluated. Based on RBT values, a second session of applanation is performed in which a second FS lamellar dissection is performed the same way as the single path profile (Fig. 11.1C).

Mixed Procedures

Arguing that the laser beam could create alterations of collagen lamellae in posterior stroma of donor corneas, FS preparation has also been combined with several mechanical procedures. Murta et al.[26] combined debulking with FS and mechanical lamellar dissection to obtain ultrathin KLE lenticules. Also, Duran et al.[27] suggested initiating posterior lamellar dissection with FS and completing it with a surgical string.

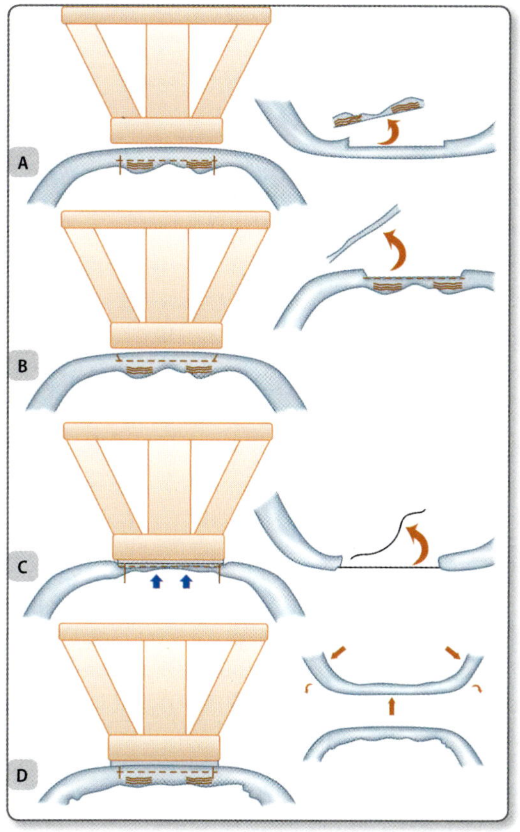

Figs 11.1A to D: (A) Cutting profiles tested with FS lasers to prepare endothelial lenticules for KLE. Lamellar dissection can be directly performed with a single or two successive lamellar cuts (horizontal red line). The lenticule is further dissected in the OR during the surgical grafting procedure; (B) To enhance smoothness of the interface, a preliminary debulking can be performed in anterior stroma; (C) Immediately followed by proceeding to the lenticule preparation; (D) Finally, lenticule preparation can be performed from the endothelial side of the cornea to lower irregularities in thickness

PREPARATION FROM ENDOTHELIAL SIDE

Femtosecond lasers are cutting with the corneal side of applanation cones as the referral plane for depth. Thus, lamellar cuts are parallel to the corneal side applied with the system regardless of the other side. Posterior collagen matrix is loose. Consequently, posterior edema can dramatically vary over the whole corneal area. This results in significant variations of lenticule thickness within the area of the lamellar cut while the referral for depth is the epithelium. Thus, lenticules were prepared from the endothelial side by using direct applanation, with or without fluid interface (Fig. 11.1D).

Each technique demonstrates some specific benefits over another. A single applanation is simple and saves time. The theoretical concern cutting from the endothelial side is toward endothelial safety, although it would provide smoother and much more regular lenticules. Anterior stromal debulking provides a compromise between different approaches (Table 11.1).

LASER SETTINGS AND OPTIMIZATION

To analyze both the efficiency of the lamellar dissection and the quality of interface, we have experimentally proceeded for ELK lenticule preparation on human corneas from eye banks. We performed either a single or a double path profile aiming to create 150 µm thick lenticules. The difficulty to dissect interface and interface smoothness were both quantified and further analyzed by scanning electron microscope (SEM). We further reproduced experiments with two different lasers, respectively running at 60 kHz and 150 kHz (IntraLase FS lasers, AMO).[28] Lasers were set as follows:

Table 11.1: Strengths and weaknesses of FS lenticules prepared with various techniques

Cutting profile	*Single/Dual lamellar cut*	*Anterior stroma debulking*	*Endothelial side*
Lamellar cut (n=)	1/2	2	1
Applanation step (n=)	1	2	1
Energy for lamellar cut	+++/++	+	+
Time consumption	+/++	+++	+
Residual bridges	+++/++	0	+
Interface smoothness	+/++	+++	++
Lenticule regularity	+/+	++	+++
Lenticule thickness	+/+	++	+++
Cutting accuracy	+/+	++	+++
Endothelial hazard	+/+	++	+++

- Running at 60 kHz: 2.4 kJ energy for lamella cut per 500-μm lamellar cut depth per 4:4 μm spot-line: step.
- Running at 150 kHz: 1.05 kJ energy for lamella cut per 500-μm lamellar cut depth per 2:2 μm spot-line: step.

Using these settings, lamellar bridges persisted in the central area (3 mm) of the lenticule (Figs 11.2A and B). The 150 kHz laser failed to generate smoother interfaces when compared to the 60 kHz laser despite settings that allowed closer spots. We concluded that interface smoothness was suboptimal using either the single or the double path profile.

To enhance smoothness of collagen lamellae at the interface of lenticules, an experiment was conducted where we debulked 350 μm of anterior stroma and performed a second lamellar cut targeting 100 μm thick lenticules from the RSB. We tested six levels of energy to perform the second lamellar cut, the goal being to obtain smooth interfaces without residual adherences and to limit the total amount of energy delivered in the vicinity of the endothelium. We controlled the quality of interfaces with 120 μm depth LASIK flap interfaces created within the anterior stroma. Within 5 minutes after the start of surgery, we observed lamellar dissections with an anterior segment OCT (Visante, Zeiss) and by SEM. Interfaces were smooth and were reproducibly easy to dissect, with FS 60 kHz lamellar cut set on: 350 μm depth, 9.0 mm diameter, 2.1 μJ, spot size/step = 4:4 for anterior stroma debulking and 150 μm depth, 8.3 mm diameter, 0.9 μJ, spot size/step = 4:4 for lenticule creation from the RSB.[29] The interface of lenticules seemed comparably smooth compared to LASIK flap interfaces (Figs 11.3A and B). However, we observed irregularities in lenticule thickness when the OCT was used. Further comparison of the lenticule's regularity after FS or mechanical procedure (Gebauer microkeratome, Germany)

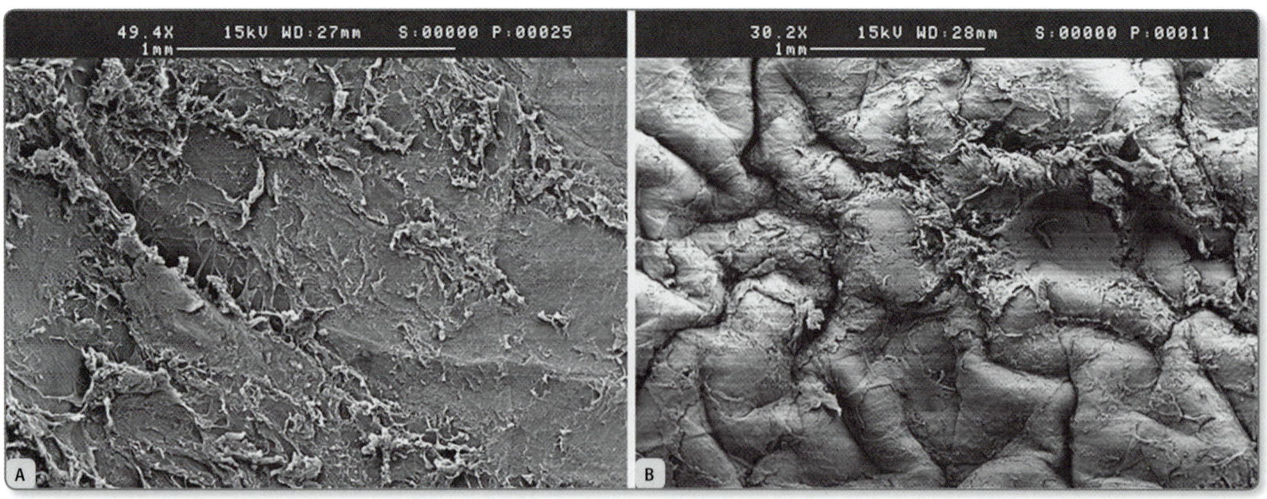

Figs 11.2A and B: Stromal interfaces of lenticules created with (A) a single or (B) a double path profile by a 60 kHz IntraLase FS. Residual collagen bridges remained in the 3 mm central area on SEM

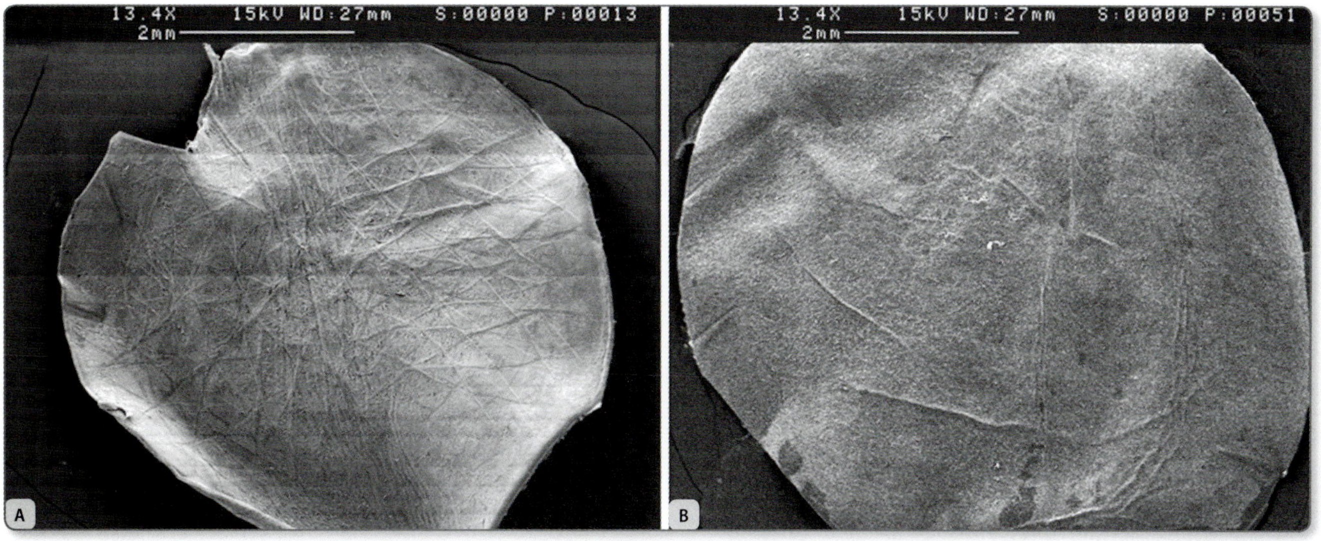

Figs 11.3A and B: Stromal interface of a lenticule created after debulking, according to the double layer procedure. Observed in SEM, the (A) stromal interface is smooth and (B) comparable to 120 µm thick LASIK flap

allowed us to conclude that higher regularity could be achieved with a microkeratome when docking from epithelial side (Figs 11.4A and B).

CLINICAL RESULTS

We prospectively followed the outcomes of patients operated on with FS-ELK for endothelial failure. We analyzed patient's visual acuities and outcomes after 6 months of follow-ups. From 2008 to 2009, we performed FS assisted ELK according to the double path profile. Data from 15 patients were analyzed in this period. From 2009 to 2012, we prepared lenticules according to the double layer profile. We did not convert any procedure. Data from 14 patients were analyzed in the period. All visual acuities improved. However, although the mean initial best visual acuity (BDVA) was poor, it did not improve dramatically after the procedure, converting from counting fingers into 20/200 with the double path technique and 20/100 with the double layer technique, respectively (Fig. 11.5). We could not obtain reliable postoperative aberrometric profiles (Wavescan, AMO), probably because of high optical disturbances. Endothelial grafts demonstrated high tendency to dislocate in the early postoperative period, whatever the preparation technique was (Table 11.2).

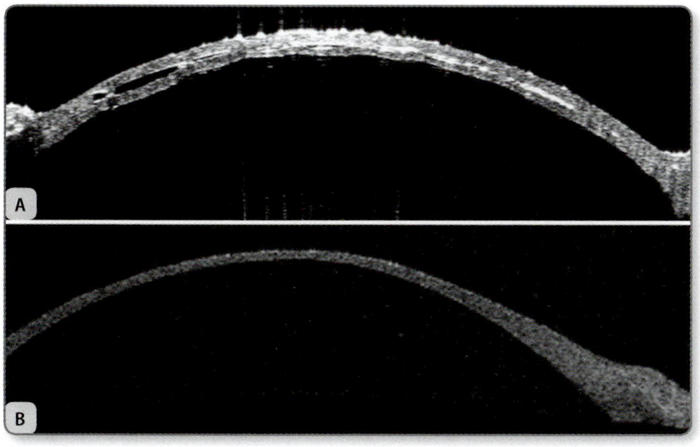

Figs 11.4A and B: Optical coherence tomography (OCT) revealed irregularity in lenticule thickness from the FS procedure docking from the (A) epithelial side whereas (B) mechanical preparation did not (Gebauer microkeratome, Germany)

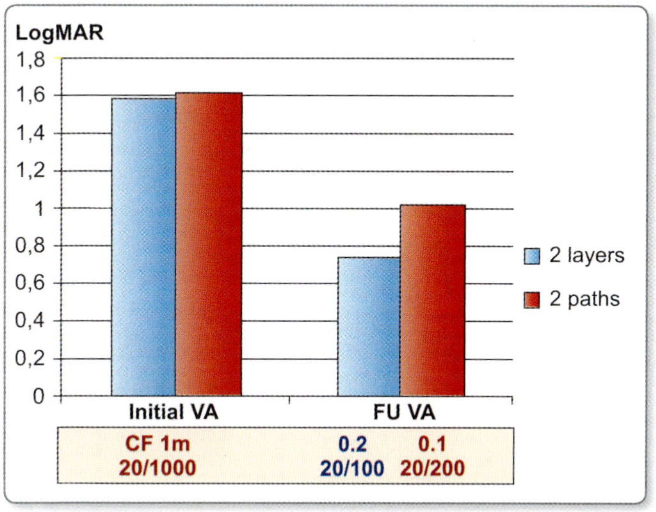

Fig. 11.5: Visual outcomes obtained with FS-assisted preparation for ELK procedures in our patients

Table 11.2: Data analyzed to approach outcomes obtained from FS-assisted ELK

	Two lamellar cuts/one step (two paths)	*Two lamellar cuts/ two steps (two layers)*
Patients (n=)	15	14
Follow-up (months)	15 (6 – 36)	11 (6 – 23)
Sex (M/F)	11/3	6/8
Date (year)	From 2008 to 2009	From 2009
Rejection (NS)	1	2
Graft dislocation (primary) (NS)	8/15	8/14

Such results argue for mechanical preparation in ELK. It is undeniable that there is still room for improvement using FS assistance in preparation of ELK button. On the other hand, any future work performed in the field is of value, considering the numerous appealing benefits demonstrated by FS assistance for corneal surgery. Some unanswered questions remain to be addressed to explain the present disappointing results. Could graft's interfaces and thickness be further improved? In the same vein, would the endothelial applanation approach be safe enough for grafts to be clinically used? Could not new on-board imaging systems help in laser beam delivery during the FS cutting phase? Are both physical characteristics of laser beam and gas emissions really neutral toward stromal cicatrization or toward primary dislocations?

CONCLUSION

Femto-assistance is not fully matured and endothelial grafts preparation is still suboptimal. Visual and surgical outcomes remain suboptimal. However, ELK procedures would greatly benefit from the numerous FS advantages, such as refractive procedures did it in the past. Both experimental research and technical improvements in femto-cataract devices are actively driving FS-assisted ELK to a reproducible and accessible procedure that, hopefully, can be performed by every ocular surgeon in the future.

REFERENCES

1. Price MO, Price FW. Descemet's stripping with endothelial keratoplasty: comparative outcomes with microkeratome-dissected and manually dissected donor tissue. Ophthalmol. 2006;113:1936-42.
2. Jones YJ, Goins KM, Sutphin JE, et al. Comparison of the femtosecond laser (IntraLase) versus manual microkeratome (Moria ALTK) in dissection of the donor in endothelial keratoplasty: initial study in eye bank eyes. Cornea. 2008;27:88-93.
3. Mootha VV, Heck E, Verity SM, et al. Comparative study of Descemet stripping automated endothelial keratoplasty donor preparation by Moria CBm microkeratome, horizon microkeratome, and IntraLase FS60. Cornea. 2010.
4. Juhasz T, Kurtz R, Raksi F, et al. The femtosecond blade: applications in corneal surgery. Optics and Photonics News. 2002;13:24-9.
5. Melles GR, Eggink FA, Lander F, et al. A surgical technique for posterior lamellar keratoplasty. Cornea. 1998;17:618-26.
6. Seitz B, Langenbucher A, Hofmann-Rummelt C, et al. Nonmechanical posterior lamellar keratoplasty using the femtosecond laser (femto-plak) for corneal endothelial decompensation. Am J Ophthalmol. 2003;136:769-72.
7. Jonas JB. Corneal endothelial transplantation using femtosecond laser technology. Eye (Lond). 2004;18:657-8.
8. Cheng YY, Pels E, Nuijts RM. Femtosecond-laser-assisted Descemet's stripping endothelial keratoplasty. J Cataract Refract Surg. 2007;33:152-5.
9. Cheng YY, Kang SJ, Grossniklaus HE, et al. Histologic evaluation of human posterior lamellar discs for femtosecond laser Descemet's stripping endothelial keratoplasty. Cornea. 2009;28:73-9.
10. Thiel MA, Kaufmann C, Dedes W, et al. Predictability of microkeratome-dependent flap thickness for DSAEK. Klin Monbl Augenheilkd. 2009;226:230-3.
11. Terry MA, Ousley PJ, Will B. A practical femtosecond laser procedure for DLEK endothelial transplantation: cadaver eye histology and topography. Cornea. 2005;24(4):453-9.
12. Javaloy J, Vidal MT, Abdelrahman AM, et al. Confocal microscopy comparison of IntraLase femtosecond laser and Moria M2 microkeratome in LASIK. Journal of Refractive Surgery (Thorofare, NJ: 1995). 2007;23:178-87.
13. Mehta JS, Shilbayeh R, Por Y-M, et al. Femtosecond laser creation of donor cornea buttons for Descemet-stripping endothelial keratoplasty. Journal of Cataract and Refractive Surgery. 2008;34:1970-5.
14. Cheng YYY, Pels E, Cleutjens JPM, et al. Corneal endothelial viability after femtosecond laser preparation of posterior lamellar discs for Descemet-stripping endothelial keratoplasty. Cornea. 2007;26:1118-22.
15. Salomao MQ, Wilson SE. Femtosecond laser in laser in situ keratomileusis. Journal of Cataract and Refractive Surgery. 2010;36:1024-32.
16. Lee JK, Nkyekyer EW, Chuck RS. Microkeratome complications. Current Opinion in Ophthalmology. 2009;20:260-3.
17. Kim JH, Lee D, Rhee KI. Flap thickness reproducibility in laser in situ keratomileusis with a femtosecond laser: optical coherence tomography measurement. J Cataract Refract Surg. 2008;34:132-6.
18. Cheng YYY, Hendrikse F, Pels E, et al. Preliminary results of femtosecond laser-assisted descemet stripping endothelial keratoplasty. Archives of Ophthalmology. 2008;126:1351-6.
19. Seery LS, Nau CB, McLaren JW, et al. Graft thickness, graft folds, and aberrations after Descemet stripping endothelial

keratoplasty for fuchs dystrophy. Am J Ophthalmol. 2012;152:910-6.

20. McLaren JW, Patel SV, Bourne WM, et al. Corneal wavefront errors 24 months after deep lamellar endothelial keratoplasty and penetrating keratoplasty. Am J Ophthalmol. 2009;147:959-65.
21. Chamberlain W, Omid N, Lin A, et al. Comparison of corneal surface higher-order aberrations after endothelial keratoplasty, femtosecond laser-assisted keratoplasty, and conventional penetrating keratoplasty. Cornea. 2012;31:6-13.
22. Koh S, Maeda N, Nakagawa T, et al. Characteristic higher-order aberrations of the anterior and posterior corneal surfaces in 3 corneal transplantation techniques. Am J Ophthalmol. 2012;153:284-90. e1.
23. Muftuoglu O, Prasher P, Bowman RW, et al. Corneal higher-order aberrations after Descemet's stripping automated endothelial keratoplasty. Ophthalmol. 2012;117:878-84.
24. Pantanelli SM, Sabesan R, Ching ST, et al. Visual performance with wave aberration correction after penetrating, deep anterior lamellar, or endothelial keratoplasty. Invest Ophthalmol Vis Sci. 2012;53(8):4797-804.
25. Yamaguchi T, Negishi K, Yamaguchi K, et al. Comparison of anterior and posterior corneal surface irregularity in Descemet stripping automated endothelial keratoplasty and penetrating keratoplasty. Cornea. 2012;29:1086-90.
26. Murta JN, Rosa A, Quadrado M, et al. Femtosecond laser and microkeratome preparation of ultrathin (UT) DSAEK grafts. The first clinical results. ARVO Meeting Abstracts. 2012;53:3136.
27. Duran JA, Grau AE, Garcia M. Femtosecond assisted technique in the donor harvesting for endothelial keratoplasty. ARVO Meeting Abstracts. 2012;53:34.
28. Rousseau A, Saragoussi J-J, Savoldelli M, et al. IntraLase endothelial keratoplasty procedure: stromal interface obtained with 60 and 150 khz lasers. ARVO Meeting Abstracts. 2011;52:742.
29. Rousseau A, Bensalem A, Garnier V, et al. Interface quality of endothelial keratoplasty buttons obtained with optimized femtosecond laser settings. Br J Ophthalmol. 2012;96(1):122-7.

Index

Page numbers followed by *f* refer to figure